THE WORK OF LIVING

THE WORK OF LIVING

Working People Talk About Their Lives and the Year the World Broke

Maximillian Alvarez

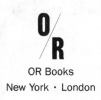

OR Books
New York · London

All rights information: rights@orbooks.com
Visit our website at www.orbooks.com

First printing 2022

Published by OR Books, New York and London

Library of Congress Cataloging-in-Publication Data: A catalog record for this book is available from the Library of Congress.

Typeset by Lapiz Digital Services.

paperback ISBN 978-1-68219-323-5 • ebook ISBN 978-1-68219-324-2

For my family

Table of Contents

Preface

I had no idea what I wanted this book to be, I just knew that it *had to be*. The COVID-19 pandemic, compounded by our government's truly villainous failure to respond adequately to it, has taken so much and so many from us. As working people, most of whom had no choice, risked—and lost—their lives keeping the gears of commerce and society turning; as many others pickled in the lonesome brine of their own homes; as time melted into a dull, endless horror, and as the horror itself became commonplace, it became clear that, regardless of what comes next, we need to keep a human record of this long moment—we need to remember how this feels. In the future, we'll need to remember how we felt about this *as it was actually happening to us*. Because those who aim to capitalize on it will tell us to remember it differently, or they'll have us recall only very select parts of the experience. The question for us then—one of the most deeply political questions of all—is: *What* will we remember, and *how* will we remember it? When the strange experience of enduring the (first) COVID-19 pandemic coagulates into history, whose voices will go on the record? Who will tell the story of what happened here? How will they tell that story? What will they focus on? And what will we care to listen to?

More importantly: How will we each see ourselves as participants in and shapers of this history? Will we forget all the things that mattered to us at the time—all the ways *we* experienced and felt about what was happening to us? Will we wash out all the raw, human stuff—the kind of stuff you'll find in this book—and leave only a clean, bloodless record of key dates and figures? Or will we carry with us the memory of something more? And will we use that memory to do good, and do better?

In case it wasn't obvious by now, I put this book together in the hope of offering a partial answer to these questions. The people and stories in this book are the kind of people and stories I think should be shaping our collective historical narrative of COVID-19; in fact, for the same reason I think it's bad and wrong to simplify, judge, and categorize people we know little about, I think we should all be deeply suspicious of any retelling of human history that leaves little room for, or deliberately excludes, the messy, complex lives of the working people who lived and made it. To see and appreciate that messiness, I believe, is the only way we can begin to understand history—and each other.

History does not happen in broad strokes, nor is it made by a few powerful people; the stories we tell about the past just make it seem that way. Living in a society that has systematically disempowered so many of us for the sake of empowering and enriching so few, it is hard to believe it's an accident that we have been taught to see history as something that certain special individuals shape and that the vast, unspecial many merely experience. I certainly hope that a viral event like the COVID-19 pandemic has made clear that the reality is always much more complex and, well, messy. True, from deadly and catastrophic decisions made (or not made) by heads of state like Donald Trump, Boris Johnson, Jair Bolsonaro, and Narendra Modi, to the decisions made (or not made) by city mayors, state governors, influential media personalities, bosses, corporate executives at pharmaceutical companies, prison wardens, etc., certain individuals *have* had a major hand in shaping the nightmarish unfolding of events—and must be held accountable for their crimes. But that is only part of the story. Each of us played a role as well. For big and small reasons—some tied to the particularities of our lives and personal histories, others to the pressures our economic realities put on us or the imprint our collective (national, local, and political) cultures leave on us—we all acted and engaged one another in certain ways over these past two years that directly contributed either to the virus spreading and hurting people or to us being able to contain it; that made it possible for us to care for each other and hold society together, or made it easier for things to fall apart. Many of us sacrificed (willingly or by force) to keep the world from collapsing, while many others took advantage of people's suffering. My point is that the deadly, contagious virus that has spread throughout the world by way of the bodies of millions of people has shown us, in the most morbidly literal way, how much of an impact we have on the world and people around us (and vice versa).

What can the history of such a world-shaking event be—how much can that history actually tell us and future generations—if it leaves no record of the kind of intimate experiences, stories, thoughts, feelings, memories, and impressions that make history human? How much can we actually understand what this pandemic was and all that it will mean for the carrying on of humanity if we relegate these things to the periphery of what's historically important? Again, I put this book together in the hope that the people, stories, and conversations in it will offer an answer: not much. This is why this book is built the way it is, why its conversations unfold the way they do—at times meandering, sometimes funny or philosophical, at other times punctured by pain and fear so deep that it hurts to read. This is also why the stories of every worker I spoke to for this book—from Kyle, a sheet metal worker in Kentucky, to Mx. Pucks, a burlesque performer and producer in Seattle, to Nick, a gravedigger in New Jersey—go way beyond the jobs they do for a living (though we talk about those, too). In the same way that I've tried from the very start of my podcast *Working People* to talk to workers not just about their jobs but about their lives— where they come from, what their families are like, what memories they hold dear, what they think about thorny political questions—I have tried to approach every conversation I recorded for this book in a way that will make it impossible for readers to ignore the whole human being behind every name tag they see, the precious life behind all the "essential work" our lives depend on.

History is messy, because it is human, and humanity is messy. The practice of history, I mean—I'm not just talking about "the past" as such. I'm talking about the stories we tell, the records we keep, and the memories we carry with us that serve as the collective lineage of our species. When we lose the beautiful human messiness of history, it becomes something else entirely, something that is not really ours, a half-true story we're told to tell about a dead past where the "significant parts" have already been colored in for us. This book aims to tell the history of this moment in a different way. Perhaps you could see it as a handful of working people, as if pushing their hands into wet concrete, pressing the imprint of their lives, thoughts, and experiences onto history before it hardens. Because they believe, as I do, that these stories are worth telling, sharing, preserving, and listening to with care. (And I'm so grateful to all of them for sharing their stories so bravely, openly, and trustingly with me. Each and every one of them is a beautiful person whom I'm honored to now know.)

That's one side of why I felt it was important to put this book together. If this book, and my work in general, ends up having any historiographical value, I hope it's for that—for preserving and defending the beautiful mess that makes history ours. On that point, though, I want to be extremely clear about something: in no way is this collection of interviews meant to be an equitably scaled or demographically and experientially representative sample of the lives of working people during the COVID-19 pandemic in the United States. If anything, one of the "big lessons" I hope readers take away from this book is that, regardless of how cliché it may sound, no two people's experiences are the same because no two people are the same. We are all, by virtue of being ourselves, unique. And that means something. As Willy Solis, a gig worker and organizer in Texas, sums up perfectly, "You can't generalize people into these big buckets and categories. Each individual person you interact with is a human being with a story, and every single story is extremely valuable."

There *are*, of course, many things and experiences that we have in common, and those things bind us together. It's what makes us understandable to and even *dependent upon* one another. And that means something, too. There are also many experiences and ways of living that are only common—or even recognizable—to certain groups of people. And there are always historical reasons for that, and sometimes those reasons involve crimes committed against our fellow humans—crimes that can never be fully undone or forgiven but can be rectified if we commit to making it so and doing it together. (Because it's the right thing to do, and because healing the wounds of history makes the world better for all of us.) If we can commit to that, if we can commit to one another, then I believe we can still find a way to live together on this planet in peace and with dignity. That's really as basic as it gets, and it shouldn't have to be such a damn far-fetched goal. It shouldn't be embarrassing to want that. To build the world we all deserve, however, means first embracing that we all still have so much to learn from and about one another.

No single conversation, and certainly no single book, can capture the totality of the beautiful mess that makes each of us who we are, nor could it faithfully "represent" the fullness and scope of our experiences of the pandemic. But I have tried to at least give that mess the respect that it—and we—deserve. Because it's there that we'll find not only the deep and true history of what happened here, but the enduring proof of what—and who—we must continue fighting for. When I was engaged in the long, painstaking process of seeking out people to interview for this book, building trust with them, talking things through, then finding time in their busy schedules to record, I tried to be as committed as possible to including a diverse range of folks working different types of jobs and living in different locations. I also, of course, sought people with a diverse range of experiences and identities—because identity is experience. And I would not have been able to make the connections I did, and this book would not exist, without the aid of friends to whom I am forever grateful: Frances Madeson, Vanessa Bain, Jeremy Waugh, Rebecca Givan, Brian "Skiff" Skiffington, Zack Pattin, Kaytlin Bailey, Bridget Huff, Lauren Kaori Gurley, Rachel Miller, and Kayla Blado.

Despite my best efforts, though, this book will be more notable for its absences than anything else—for the people and stories not in it. I certainly did the best I could, given the constraints: that we are still living in a pandemic, and people are stressed out, distanced, and terrified; that, for most of 2020, it felt like the fate of the country was hanging in the balance of a relentlessly depressing election, and people were anxiously focused on that; that, even with the money I could pay out of my pocket for their time, it was a lot to ask anyone to take this huge step and give so much of themselves to someone they had never met. Accepting that this book was always going to be chronically incomplete does little to soften the shame. But it should be a vital reminder that no book, no podcast, no one project, and no one person can ever fulfill the burningly necessary task of sharing and listening to the stories of our fellow workers—and doing so in a way that dignifies their lives and honors their humanity. It should remind us that there is an entire universe of human experience beyond the cages of our own heads. Every day you walk down the street, you are passing by an endless, living archive of stories and memories, wisdom and pain, joy and need, and a deep, boundless yearning to be heard. And everyone deserves to be heard. While providing only an extremely limited view into the lives of others, I hope that *The Work of Living* serves as a reminder that the complexity and uniqueness of every human soul is as much of a miracle to behold and cherish and defend as the world itself. It is unjust and unbearable to live in a society that makes so little room for stories like these to get the attention and respect they deserve, and I hope we are all moved to do something about that.

That is all to say, I hope that what is painfully missing from this book is found in the work of others. Whether it involves striking up conversations with our coworkers and our neighbors, sitting down and listening (really listening) to our family members, or opening up spaces to connect with strangers, we should recognize that this work is important—and that it will take *all* of us to do it.

This brings us to the other side—the much bigger and perhaps more significant side—of why I put this book together. I did it for a deeply human reason, which is to say, a deeply political reason.

Honoring the humanity of working people has been the singular guiding aim for my work as a podcaster, writer, and activist. On the most elemental level, I do this work because I have a deep love for the working class; because I am dedicated to the cause of ensuring that everyone can live a comfortable, joyful, free, and dignified life; and because I share the conviction that everyone deserves to feel heard and seen, to feel that their lives and their stories *matter*. I believe we owe that to one another. On a political level, I do this work because building bonds of solidarity between members of an incredibly diverse working class is vital to creating a grassroots movement that will have the strength and staying power to ensure workers get the justice, dignity, and livable planet that we all deserve.

Connecting with one another on our most human levels is essential to building this kind of solidarity. It is much easier to feel common cause with others once you recognize that they are just as human as you are, that their lives and their ways of being in the world are more closely connected to your own than you previously thought. It is essential, moreover, to forging a shared sense of justice. It is much easier to feel angry about the exploitation and dehumanization of others once you look past their job title or uniform and see people—people with families, histories, and dreams—who hurt just as much as you do. That is precisely why we are so routinely discouraged and distracted from connecting with one another in these ways. As I once wrote for the magazine *Current Affairs*, "In a world where working people are consistently reminded that we don't matter, where we become accustomed to being, at best, exploitable and, at worst, invisible to each other, seeing and affirming the trembling humanity we share with our neighbors is revolutionary."

The wilds of twenty-first-century capitalism, and the hard lives it forces so many of us to live, have gotten us so used to being dehumanized—denied our most basic needs and desires for purpose, connection, comfort, and joy—and so used to being alienated from one another, that we must collectively commit to doing the patient, tender work of finding each other again (or for the first time). We must listen to each other and remind ourselves of that which life under capitalism forces us to forget: that we're all human, and we all deserve better than this.

The interviews in this book have been edited for clarity and readability, although every effort has been made to keep the text faithful to speakers' individual word choices and speech patterns.

1. Nick Galuppo

My name is Nick. I reside in central-northern New Jersey—it used to be a smaller suburb, but I guess you could say things have picked up in terms of speed and people. I'm thirty-eight years old. Been working in a cemetery almost two decades now.

When I was eighteen, I was working at a seasonal job unloading trucks and got laid off. Now, my father was a union carpenter, as was his older brother, and his father before him. I figured I'd go into the construction outfit as a laborer, maybe like a journeyman or something. But I seen how my father lived—he was laid off a lot, he was traveling all over the place—and I didn't like that inconsistency of work, you know? So, I kind of had . . . I guess you could say I had a bit of reluctance about it.

And one night, he was at the Knights of Columbus talking to a friend. He said, "Hey, my son's looking for work. If anybody hears anything, knows anything, keep your ears open." And one guy there responded and said, "Hey, I'm a regional manager for seven cemeteries," and these were cemeteries from North Jersey, South Jersey, Delaware, Rhode Island—like, over three different states. He said, "The work's hard, the work's messy, but if the kid don't mind working, we'll give him a shot."

So, I got the job. This was in 2001–2002. When I started, I was put on a ninety-day probationary period. I was only told I'd be staying-on on my eighty-ninth day—this was on Christmas Eve, about five minutes before quitting time . . .

Max: [Laughs.]

Nick: The manager was . . . everything you'd expect him to be. He was a ruthless little guy. Little in every sense of the word: morally, physically, mentally. He was a little egomaniac. But what are you gonna do? He was a boss, he was strict, etc., and that's fine.

So, like I said, I got the job. And I'm nineteen years old at the time—very wet behind the ears. And, shit, at that point, I wasn't even really driving much. I didn't have a lot of money then, and car insurance is expensive. But it was around that time I got my first vehicle and started working in the cemetery. It was nothing like I thought it was gonna be. I was told it was like a landscaping job—you know, "You're gonna cut grass, you're gonna rake leaves." Like some sort of a Parks Department gig. Couldn't be farther from the truth . . . It's a death factory. It's busy, like a construction site. It's like a fast-paced construction site . . . for the dead.

As far as the places that I work in—there's three cemeteries in a small area. We're responsible for two of them, as per the contract that we just negotiated. So, we got the two of them. One is a mainly Jewish cemetery, close to three hundred acres in size, which does about 1,500 burials a year. It's open seven days a week. And, you know . . . it really is wild. You got so many different elements that come into play that make the job different from the aforementioned construction site. With construction, you got mom-and-pop shops or you got commercial construction. But either way, you've still got some oversight: You have state laws, federal guidelines, you have OSHA [Occupational Safety and Health Administration], you have all these different levels of bureaucracy and regulation.

It's different in the cemetery, though. The cemetery is kind of like everybody's best-kept secret. Everybody knows that you die. But nobody really understands what happens when you die or how that process comes to be.

Now, that process can vary based on your religion, based on how you want to get buried, or interred, or entombed, or cremated. Things can vary quite a bit. But in my experience, which is almost two decades in a high-volume location, what's known as a "Tier One" location, when you take the geography of where I work, the varying soil content, the manner in which people are buried, the water table—you mix all that up with how many people get buried in such a tight area, it's a recipe for chaos.

People might think, "Oh, you work in a cemetery? You must be coming out with a lantern and a shovel at midnight to bury somebody peacefully on a hill, under the moonlight." Yeah, it's not like that at all. It's, um, it's pretty wild.

Max: Damn, man. I bet. And I definitely want to dig into all of this with you. I mean . . . no pun intended.

Nick: [Laughs.] There ya go.

Max: I was just thinking about you as a young man. You said you kind of fell into this job—and you were only nineteen at the time! I can only imagine what my dumbass nineteen-year-old self would have done in that situation. So, I'm curious to know: Were you a more adventurous type? I feel like you'd kind of have to be if you're the type of person who says, "Sure, let's do it!" when you're offered that job, right? Or did you have some sort of closer relationship with death and cemeteries growing up that you think made you more capable of sticking with this work than other people would be?

Nick: I wouldn't say I had any particular experiences with death that made me more capable. I'll say this, though: My father—he worked for a living, and he worked hard for a living. He had hands like cinder blocks. He was on the road at five in the morning, he'd get home around five, six at night. At ten he'd go to the bar, wherever he was bartending—get home around three in the morning. And I watched him . . . My father had a lot of fortitude. He was a pretty strong-willed guy. And when I got the job he said to me, "Nick, I put my name on that, so you gotta do the right thing. You gotta man up out there." He didn't really know what the job entailed, but he knew that I could definitely handle the job physically. But as far as handling the job mentally and emotionally? That was always going to be a toss-up. At the end of the day, though, he knew that I couldn't soil his name or his reputation. And I knew I couldn't do that. So, that's what led me to just stick my nose into it and say, "I gotta move forward. Can't take any steps backward. I just gotta man up and do this."

And when I got there—it was funny, because I'm the young guy there. And you got people who'd been there a little while, and you got jokers who would be like, "Oh, you haven't seen nothing yet, you're just a puppy. Wait till you see this, wait till you do that . . ." And I rose to that occasion, to that challenge. I've earned quite the reputation for being like a roll-your-sleeves-up-and-just-get-into-it kind of guy out there. But I'll tell you this:

Fifteen years ago, what I was doing . . . it didn't register or resonate with me at all. It was a job. It was simply a job. Some days it's raining, there's four inches of rain over eight hours, but you still gotta open up graves (and we'll get into that part of it a little bit later). You still gotta deal with all of that.

But now, mentally, it has a different impact as I've gotten older and I've watched people I know die, and as I've realized myself, "Hey, wow, what do you know? I'm not this young, immortal guy anymore." I got gray hair, I got wrinkles—I'm getting slower, getting weaker, no matter how much I try to fight it. I'm digging people's graves . . . in due time, I'm digging mine, too. But if you're going to risk living, you have to risk dying. It just comes with the territory.

What's funny is—well, not funny, but oddly enough, on my first burial . . . and, like I said, I've done 1,500 a year, on average, for eighteen, nineteen years . . . I know the kid's name. I know his first name, know his last name. I know how he passed, because it had an impact on me. He wasn't much younger than I was at the time. A season later, his father died. Year after that, the grandfather died. Three generations of men, dead, just like that. And I remember being there at that first burial and seeing the mother. At the time she was, let's just say, early thirties. Beautiful woman, long black hair, distraught. I saw her two, three years later, and her hair was white as a ghost. In around nine hundred days, she looked like she had aged sixty years. I saw it then, but it didn't affect me. Not until about a decade and a half later. It just started to sink in. It's weird how all the other things that I've physically seen and experienced . . . and I've done *a lot*, I've been on the front of it my entire career there. It hasn't been until the last, I'd say, four or five years . . . I guess, maybe, as the brain matures, or as your own mortality starts to creep in . . . it's just like, every day, these things become more real.

When I was twenty, though, it was no big deal. The biggest deal for me was, "Am I gonna have to work later than I'm supposed to? Are they gonna tell me I have to work Saturday or Sunday?" You know what I mean? I'm a kid, I want to go out on the weekends, enjoy my life. Now it's different. I feel like somebody's gotta do this work, and I try to do the best I can. I take pride in that. I mean, it's definitely an old ritual, right? People have been burying people as long as we've been doing anything else. It's the thing that separates us from the animals: We bury each other. But at the same time, I'm saying to myself, "Shit, man." Because doing this work—I robbed myself of that idea of peace, that tranquility of final resting places when people go visit a loved one . . . I don't have that. I don't have that for myself, I don't have that for people I know or people I try to console. It's just gone. That was the trade that I made when I started working as a gravedigger for a living.

Max: Well, shit, I can imagine! Because, like you said, this is like society's best kept secret—it's the thing that we all know is waiting for us, but we do our best to not really think about it until we actually have to. Even now, I'm thinking about where I grew up back home, in Southern California. We lived down the road from a cemetery where I had family members buried. For most of my life it was just part of the landscape. It was a nice, quiet, gated, manicured-lawn type of place where people would come to pay their respects. There was a kind of tranquility to the whole scene. But it wasn't until later in life that I realized that this kind of tranquility doesn't just happen. It's a product that is made by workers like you—workers who have to see all of the non-tranquil stuff, workers whose job is to create that sort of atmosphere for the loved ones of the deceased. It's like everything else in this world, in this economy, this capitalist way of living. Workers like you make a sort of product for us to consume, but one of the main requirements is that we don't see or think about all the labor that goes into that. We don't see everything you go through on a day-to-day basis. It's almost like an essential part of your job is to keep people from seeing what you see.

Nick: Yes, yes. Well put.

Max: I want to ask you more about that work you do on a day-to-day basis and the process that goes into creating this kind of atmosphere for people. But before we get there, I wanted to take a quick step back and try to put myself back in your shoes when you were nineteen years old. It sounds like you didn't envision yourself becoming a professional gravedigger, but having watched your dad go from job to job, it seems like, more than anything, you were looking for something that was just more stable?

Nick: Yes, absolutely. My father—he worked two jobs for most of his life. There was three of us at home and my mother didn't work. She's a good woman but has mental issues and battles with stuff like depression. So, my father was at the forefront. Like I said, he was a journeyman: He would travel to an area, work for six months; it would be feast or famine, basically. There'd be times when he was working and maybe the overtime just wasn't there. So, now he's coming home from one job and then he'd be tending bar down the road, at a place that his godparents owned, a place that his father helped build when he came home from World War II. And this place, what used to be a community hub, had turned into a place of violence—bikers and gangs, this and that. So, I'd see this guy, my father, who built foundations for a living—I'd see this guy come home with his hands split open twenty different ways from working with concrete ten to twelve hours a day, put his gear down, just to go back out to tend bar. And then he'd come home covered in blood or something—maybe somebody got shot, somebody got stabbed, or whatever. So, yeah, the consistency of the work wasn't there. Then one day my father says to me, "Hey, Nick, this job's just five minutes down the road." He put things in perspective for me—like, right away, that just made a lot of sense.

Speaking of that, the first couple years into this job, I was actually offered work from a good friend of mine. He said, "Hey, I got a job for you in the port. My girlfriend's father loves you, you got such a good work ethic—you're in. You can make three times what you're making in the cemetery. It's not laborious." And his girlfriend's father came to me and said, "Nick, I've been here a long time, I can get you this, get you that. That cemetery job is a dead-end gig." I said to him, "Hey, I appreciate that, man. I really do. But I'm good." Part of me regrets it, because you have the financial aspect, the physical aspect—would have been a lot more money, would have been easier. I would have traveled to the same place every day. But at the same time, it's almost like I'm tied to this now. This might sound incredibly cliché, but I gotta tell you: I can't envision myself really doing much else. You know? Not that I wouldn't *want* to. But it just . . . it's almost like a burden to endure. That's what it is. And don't get me wrong: I'm not trying to say we're special, because we're not. There are people in this world who do important stuff—people who save people's lives, people who advance technology. We're not saving anything; we're the opposite.

But it's essential. There's a need for it. So, there's a burden that I feel like I almost have to endure, and that's the job. I just really don't see myself doing anything else.

Max: Let's talk about that, that sense that this is where you're supposed to be and that this is the work you're meant to do. I want to know more about how that developed. I know you said that when you started at the cemetery you were on a ninety-day probationary period. What was that like? Like you said, you were going into this green and you were expecting it to be more of a landscaping gig, and that you were dead wrong about that . . .

Nick: [Laughs.] Yeah.

Max: Let's go back to those first ninety days, then. Put yourself back there: What were you doing? What were you seeing? And how was it all changing you in the process?

Nick: Well, I get there, and my boss says, "Go over there, hop in the truck with that guy, and he's gonna show you what's up." So, I get in the truck with this guy. "How you doing?" he says. "My name is Ed." I asked him what we were gonna be doing and he goes, "Oh, you're gonna be on a burial crew with me. You're gonna be driving the dump truck." I said, "What the hell is that?" "Well," he says, "this is a cemetery, dude. We bury people. And new guys like you, if they make the job, they want to break you in. You're gonna be the ground man for a backhoe operator." He tells me to just sit back and watch for these first couple days. "After that," he tells me, "there's going to be expectations you're gonna need to meet if you're going to work here." This guy is still a friend of mine—very intelligent guy. He probably could have done anything. But for whatever reason, he chose to stay here. The key word there is "intelligent." He's intelligent. I'm not. I know why I stayed; I don't know why he stayed.

So, basically, there's three sectors of the job. You *do* have landscaping— back then, that was reserved for part-time work. Now it's known as work that's "subcontracted out" by other companies: They subcontract the leaf cutting, grass cutting, etc. Then you have other stuff that the full-time guys do, and that's burials, that's monument installations, plaque installations, etc. But the burial crew is a three-sector job: You have a boards division, a setup division, and then you have a digging division. And each crew is a pair of two guys. If you get busy, obviously, and if you have the manpower, they'll tag more people in.

My first week was observing. And then, within the second or third day, I was learning how to carry a casket and how to get somebody's loved one from a hearse to the grave site. While that sounds simple, it's not. A lot of times in the movies you'll see six, seven, eight guys carrying a metal box with handles on the side, and they're carrying it over a flat piece of ground, and they put it over this hole in the ground in this wide-open green pasture . . . nuh-uh. It's you and another guy: One guy's carrying the head, walking backward, one guy's carrying the feet, walking forward. And you've gotta, like, sidestep to get the casket in a really, really tight area.

In those first ninety days I had to learn how to operate a Ford F-550. And when I say "operate," I mean: You gotta be able to drive that truck in reverse the way you can drive it going forward. You gotta be able to back that thing up within inches of your target in this rat maze of super tight areas. And, like I said, you're moving monuments, you're all over the place . . . it's a rat race that exists within this little world. You have to learn how to operate a lot of different equipment in a short period of time. There's a lot of labor involved to get these people in the ground.

Every section of every block in these cemeteries is different and unique unto themselves. There's different areas that require liner installation. Some people just go into a quarter-inch pine box in the ground. You might have to move ten to fifteen headstones just to get in and dig a grave with a backhoe, and you have to get all the dirt out. There's a lot of stuff involved. But there's no real, like, OSHA oversight. It's almost like a little farm. You got equipment from like the '50s and '60s and it's all jerry-rigged, and you just gotta learn on the fly how to become very intimate with this equipment and use it properly. Because if you don't, you're gonna hurt somebody, you're gonna hurt yourself, or, worse, you could get permanently injured or killed. Or, excuse my language, you're gonna really fuck up somebody's last ride—for them and for their family. So, yeah, there's a lot to it.

Like I said, my first week was just learning the bare minimum so they could inject me into the rotation and have me serve the purpose that I'm supposed to serve there. And I'm doing all that while under the scrutiny of management, and the employees who are tasked with training me—and then you also have rabbis and hundreds of people present, because you're performing all of this in front of people. And obviously people are extremely emotional and, you know, people's customs and perspectives vary from religion to religion. Even in the Jewish community there's different factions, different ways of practicing that religion for different sects of that religion. You gotta memorize this stuff, you gotta know this stuff and become intimate with it, because you gotta meet these people's demands and wishes. And you gotta do this within a very small time frame.

If I was to paint you a picture . . . You get to work at 7:30 in the morning, and you get handed a burial sheet. That burial sheet might say: "10:45 Block, 11-B, 26 by 81, menorah"; "11:00 Block, 12-A, 22 by 75, Bloomfield Cooper"; "1:00–1:30 . . ." And that burial sheet—those are people who are going in the ground by that time frame. So, if it says "1:00" and it's 7:30, then there's an 11:45 and a 12:30 and a 1:00—you gotta have those graves ready and open and available by the time these people come. Then, we have until nine o'clock at night for funeral homes to call in and schedule other funerals. Because in the Jewish religion, people go in the ground before sundown. If someone dies in the morning and they want to have a burial by ten, eleven o'clock, they're gonna do that. Now, some of them wait till the next day, but they're gonna go in the ground before sundown the next day. It's just a very packed, tight schedule. And it gets crazy, man . . . it really does.

There are a lot of aspects that make this job unique and different from your traditional memorial park, which is where everything is flat and there's markers installed in the ground. At my cemetery, they're all upright monuments, they're all custom, they're different sizes, they're on single foundations in a wet area with different soil content. The areas are very unstable. You risk cave-ins, which could mean loss of monument, loss of foundation, loss of remains, or worse. You yourself risk death while you're inside these trenches tying these areas back. It's a very tough job. Nobody's embalmed, the areas are very wet, people are not buried very deep. It's a very fragile process. And it's something that people don't ever really shed a lot of light on. And, you know, the things that you see . . .

I could tell them to you and you probably wouldn't believe it. But it's true, nonetheless.

If you take a quarter-inch pine box, and you put a human inside that, and they're not embalmed . . . that box is made to break down, it's made to decompose, because that is in accordance with this person's religious traditions. But most people don't understand that. They understand that different religions have different processes for burials, but they don't understand *the process*. And you don't want to be the one to explain it. For example, say you have two hundred people coming to a grave; twenty to thirty of them are close family, and they're very distraught. Somebody might say to you, "This is the wrong grave! This isn't right." Now, you know for a fact that it's the right grave, because there's a system put in place where we lay out graves and there's mapping and all this stuff that goes into it. But there are a number of reasons why they don't think it's the right one. Let's just use one of the variables: Their monument was moved. We moved it so it wasn't in the way and we could dig the grave. And not only that—it was moved because the grave next to it from a year prior has caved in and destabilized. That grave is completely gone. So, the family gets to the grave, distraught, and they see a bunch of monuments and headstones that were originally placed in one spot have been moved; they see muddy tire tracks everywhere, the area's all torn up; they had a grave that was there and intact with plantings and bushes a year ago, and now it's gone. And they're distraught because they just lost their family member. And you have to explain to them, "Well, no, ma'am, no, sir . . . that monument was moved to excavate the burial site, but it's going to go back at our earliest convenience. And the grave to the right—the planting's gonna get replaced but, unfortunately, the ground caved in." And then somebody might ask, "What are those metal bars?" Because, in accordance with that religion, people aren't supposed to get buried with anything metal, anything that doesn't break down. And that is true, which is why those bars in the ground are temporary. What you don't want to tell them is that those metal bars are made to hold back the loved one who went in the ground a year prior, to keep them from rolling into the next grave that you're putting the person in today.

But you don't want to explain that to people, you know? What you end up doing is you try to hide that from them, not because you're doing anything wrong, but because you almost want to protect them from their own questions. And you do it to give them the peace of mind that you no longer have.

The fact of the matter is this is the most time-efficient, optimal way of doing this type of work. You might have state law regulations, or OSHA will say, "Anything four feet or deeper needs a trench box"—one of those metal frames you put in the grave when you're digging to prevent cave-ins. But you *can't* put a trench box in there; it's not practical. Trench boxes don't adjust to these sizes, so you put in shale bars, you tie the graves back. There's all these different variables—there's just so much to it. This is the process that I stepped into when I took the job. When you start, you inherit the process, and your job is to mimic that process to the best of your abilities. In certain cases, you could make the process better, so long as you're allowed to. But there ain't no other way: People are getting buried out there; it's a practice that's been going on for thousands of years, and they want to continue it. But they're not getting buried in the dry sands of the Middle East; they're getting buried in an area that was wet farmland or marsh eighty years ago, and now it's all filled up. The whole area is just a wet bowl of clay in certain parts where the water doesn't drain, or it's wet sand. Try digging a rectangular hole and keeping it that shape on a wet beach—it's not possible. And yet, people are getting buried in sandy, wet areas, not unlike the beach.

But with the way these cemeteries are—they're businesses, after all— they don't lay out any real borders: People are buried next to each other with not even an inch to spare. It's incredible the way people get buried . . . it's incredible. You have natural water tables, you have different soil contents, like we discussed, then you have all these monuments that are granite. Granite is four times heavier than concrete per square foot. So, you have one of the heaviest naturally occurring materials being installed all over the place, like a set of dominoes, on top of a very unstable ground. Then you gotta get massive amounts of equipment and humans to that area to excavate and basically destabilize these areas, and the people resting there in peace, in order to provide this service for the next person. And you might have a two-hour window to get that done and make sure the other five are done so you can be ready to come back and backfill those graves when the people aren't there.

It's a rat-race construction site with blood-borne pathogens and extremely bad conditions. On a regular construction site, when it rains, you shut the job down. When you're doing a roofing job and there's a foot of snow, you're not roofing. With us, it's business as usual. When it's 110 degrees and everybody else is taking a heat break, you still gotta bury people.

Like I said, there's all these different factors that come into play. And when you add those up with the economy and the way things have been going in our country, what you have now is a lack of equipment and a lack of manpower to perform these same services, so it puts an even bigger burden and more stress on the individual—if they care about what they're doing. I've been doing this half my life, and I'm not that old, so I do care. It's . . . it's a bag to carry, Max. It really is . . .

Max: I mean, I can genuinely only imagine . . .

Nick: . . . getting splashed in the face with human remains. It happens all the time—very common. And it's just business as usual.

Max: Jesus. I'm trying to imagine this, and I'm trying to use bits and pieces from my limited life experience to understand what you're describing to me. There's one memory, in particular, that comes to mind. I would say about nine to ten years ago, I was working as a temp in factories and warehouses back in Southern California. This was when the recession and the "recovery" were still really bad and it was really hard to find work. I would just go to this temp agency at like three to four in the morning and wait for an assignment. Some of the jobs were really easy—well, not "easy," but very straightforward. They would just send you to this or that warehouse, and your job was to move those boxes onto that pallet, wrap them up, put them on a truck, easy peasy. But there was one assignment in particular that no one wanted to get. I distinctly remember one day I was sitting in this cheap, rundown, strip-mall-temp-agency waiting room at like 4:15 in the morning, which is the only time in Southern California when it's actually cold. It was still dark out. I remember I had a shitty cup of 7-Eleven coffee in my hand, and I was trying to read a book to stay awake. I remember these guys coming into the agency from an assignment they had been on, and they were yelling in Spanish. I could only hear bits and pieces of what they were saying, but they kept saying that they wouldn't go back to this job because of "el olor" (the smell). Then I heard things like "sangre" (blood). The smell of blood. I couldn't quite piece together what they were yelling about, but I got a crash course, man, because then the woman behind the desk calls my name, and she says, "Okay, here's your assignment, it's a fifteen-minute drive away. You better get going." So, I drove to this factory, and the purpose of this factory was to have us dressed in full, almost like hazmat gear, and work in the bowels of this steam-filled hell. And what we had to do was sift through and sort out these endless piles of dirty laundry from hospitals in the area.

Nick: Right.

Max: If we pulled out a smock, we would have to put those in one bin. If we pulled out a blanket, we had to put those in another bin. I came to understand what those men back in the temp agency were complaining about. The smell is something that still haunts me. Because it's like you said, just like at the cemetery: When you go to a hospital to visit a loved one, they try to keep it as clean and calm as possible, but all of the unclean stuff still has to go somewhere. We were working in the place where most of it ended up. There were all kinds of human remains stained on the hospital laundry, and it was our job to make it all clean again and send it back. Guys would run off the line because they couldn't handle the smell; they would leave, throw up, and never come back. Thankfully, I only worked at that place for a short amount of time before I was reassigned to another warehouse. But I remember working next to one guy there—we were standing next to each other in the laundry-picking line. Older Black guy, maybe in his fifties—he was one of the few people there who wasn't a temp. He'd been working there for years. I remember him just saying to me at one point, "Yeah, the smell doesn't bother me anymore," and he talked me through it. Hearing you talk, I could almost hear his voice again. I remember him telling me, "You're only gonna survive here if you take it seriously. If you can get past the initial revulsion, you'll see how necessary this work is." Then he told me, "Put some shit in your nose, or put some Vicks on your upper lip, so the smell doesn't overwhelm you."

You said it yourself that this is all the kind of stuff that no one wants to see, but it's the stuff you and your coworkers have to deal with every day. Could you talk a little more about that? What is it like adjusting to these conditions, all the things you see, and trying not to be affected by it? Well, *obviously* you're going to be affected by it, but how do you learn to live with it and carry on for years, even decades?

Nick: When I first started, this was maybe eight or nine months in, the other guys saw that I was the type of kid who . . . I guess they saw that I had that ability to just push on and deal with it. They said, "Oh, man. Just wait till you get *this*—you're not gonna believe it." I said, "What?" They said, "Disinterment." "What's that?" Well, after people get buried, sometimes their family moves and they want to take their loved ones with them. So, I did a disinterment one day. We were in a nice, dry, sandy area, and we took this person out of the ground who had been there for ten years. We took the casket, put it in a bigger casket, put it on a vault truck and shipped it away. No big deal. I said to these guys, "This is nothing." They said, "Wait till you get a bad one."

Then, one day, we get a disinterment in a wet area where it's all clay. The person's only been in the ground for like six months, but the box is destroyed already from the weight of the clay—and they're not embalmed. And there's not really any, like, PPE [Personal Protective Equipment] or any of the things we're talking about—hazmat suits and stuff like that. You can get a pair of leather gloves or something, or you could shove some Vicks or a scarf in your nose if you want. I never did. I just wanted to be *that* guy, you know? But this was when I was younger. So, we're taking this person out of a very wet area; the water doesn't really have anywhere to go—it's in the clay—and the person's only been in the ground for a little bit of time. So, it's . . . it's bad, man. It's very bad. You see things and you smell things, and you're essentially wearing it: You're up to your elbows in the decomposition fluids of somebody . . . or someone who used to be somebody.

When I was younger, I took pride in it not bothering me. Now, I almost feel guilty in a way. After years of doing this job, just going and going and going—I'm professional, I'm calculated, it does not bother me. There's no flinching, there's no gagging, there's just doing the job, getting it done.

Then you go home, and maybe you don't think about it that day—maybe it'll be tomorrow, maybe next week . . . but that guilt just starts to set in. That's the only way I can describe it; that's the only emotion I can point to. I just harbor this guilt. And I don't know why or where the guilt comes from. It's not like *I* caused this. I'm just trying to do my job. Maybe the guilt comes from the fact that it doesn't affect me physically—it doesn't move me that way. It does for a lot of people, and I understand that. For me, it doesn't. Now, mentally, emotionally . . . that's selective. When I see somebody who's ninety years old, I'm like, "God bless 'em. They lived a good life. They had a good run." But when it's a kid who got hit by a car, or cancer takes somebody prematurely, or whatever, then it just knocks the wind out of you. It sticks to you, like you stepped in gum, and it's just stuck to you for a while. Now, the more you walk, the more you wear that gum off your shoe, the more you can get away and escape. But that depression really hangs on you, like a weight. But physically? Yeah, maybe my guilt comes from it not having the impact on me that it should. Or maybe it's the guilt from knowing that when I say "I'm sorry" to someone I know who's lost someone, *I* know that *they* know. Because I've explained the process to them—they're interested and will ask me about it—and I've essentially taken away that peace that they would have had. Maybe that's where the guilt comes from.

I couldn't imagine what our military family—what these people deal with. Because they're forced to take a life, defend theirs, defend somebody else's, and then deal with everything—like the guilt—that comes with that. And I'm not trying to compare what I do to what they do. I'm just trying to make the correlation to explain that feeling of guilt.

There are people who can work in a cemetery for a long time and never deal with anything remotely close to the stuff we've been talking about. Had you spoken to a gravedigger in a small Catholic cemetery, I could tell you for a fact they wouldn't be talking about any of this, because things differ so much depending on where you are. Where I am, you got a couple of different religious groups with specific customs, and there's a cause and effect to that. You mix that with the water tables, the varying soil contents, and the amount of people we put in the ground—it really intensifies the whole experience. And . . . it's weird, man. I've always wanted to be able to talk to somebody about what I've experienced, because my experiences are extremely rich and vast, and there's a lot of them. I appreciate you giving me the opportunity to speak on this.

Max: Well, I want to thank *you* for sharing so openly with me, man. I'm honestly just kind of blown away by all this. I want to talk to you about how things have been for you and your coworkers and the communities you serve during the COVID-19 pandemic. But before we get there, I'm thinking about the way you described that guilt that just starts to stick to you—like gum on your shoe, I think, is how you put it. I'm also thinking about how, going back to what we were saying before, workers at these cemeteries, like yourself, are going through such intense work—physically, emotionally, psychologically—to create that peace, or the illusion of peace, for people who want to send their loved ones off the right way. That really struck me, and it reminded me of this book I read about the Civil War: I think it's called *This Republic of Suffering* by Drew Gilpin Faust. She talks about how the Civil War in the U.S. was like this earth-shattering moment when an entire population was forced to reckon with the reality of mass death. And she makes a really interesting connection there. Because, as she describes in the book, at the same time that the Civil War was happening—and so many young men were dying and getting their limbs blown off with cannons and guns, and so much horrifying stuff was happening—you also had the emergence of photography. You had all these families from the North and the South who were praying that, if their loved ones died, they would go to heaven as whole human beings—they'd find eternal peace in the afterlife, in the kingdom of God.

Nick: Right.

Max: But it was very hard for a lot of people to square that, to maintain this vision of a peaceful afterlife, when they would *see* photographs of their loved ones and other soldiers just literally blown to bits. It kind of shattered the illusion that they needed—the illusion of their loved ones dying and resting peacefully. Because they got to see, through photographs, the real carnage of the battlefield. And it really fucked with their understanding of what happens to people, to souls, after they die. I bring that up because, like . . . we don't ever have that sort of reckoning on a mass scale.

All of that weight falls on you and your coworkers. But for the larger public, it's like we try really hard to maintain this fiction and keep all the gory counter-evidence out of sight.

Nick: That's well said, man. It's been a long time since America has experienced the extremely visceral and tangible violence of mass death or tragedy. People are really disconnected from it, from the chaos. I had a grandmother who passed away from diabetes. Before she died they took a toe, they took a foot, they took a limb, and then eventually she passed. I didn't give no thought to this at the time—I was a kid. But then, one day, I got the manager saying to me, "Hey, listen, when you're digging that hole over there, make sure you're careful, cuz we gotta find a leg." And I'm like, "Ah, shit." So, now I'm sifting through the soil, trying to find this limb from the knee down in a medical bag that someone had just tossed in there, in the grave next to the one I'm digging, before covering it over with dirt. Like I said, this work definitely takes that peace away from you. I think that, for people who are religious, this job will either bring them closer to their faith, or it'll shoot them farther away, but you're definitely not just gonna idle in the same spot. Same for people who don't have that religious perspective: You're either gonna go more left or more right. You're gonna get closer or you're gonna move farther away; but there's no hovering in the same area and keeping the same perspective. That's impossible.

I wasn't a religious person growing up, and I wouldn't consider myself religious now. But I would say that I definitely pray more. I am definitely thankful for peace, for the peace that people I love and care about experience, and I pray that we can all just maintain that. Because seeing it up close, living and dealing with it—it really puts things into perspective for me. How important is making more money a year? How important is it to have a nicer place, a nicer car, or whatever? Scratch that, man. I don't care about that anymore. It just doesn't matter to me. I want to provide for my son and make sure that he's educated, that he's got hot meals, clothing, and all the necessities. But I'm not about all that extra stuff that would usually drive somebody in this capitalist society—going from zero to one thousand, going up and back down. I just want to get through my day, come home, and spend time with the people I love. Because I realize: Absolutely, life is limited. Absolutely, it's over at any moment. Absolutely, we're not in control of it. You can't slow it down, you can't speed it up—we have no say over it. If you're going to risk living, you have to do it at the cost of knowing that this shit is temporary. You're gonna die, and you're gonna wind up just like him, her, him, or whoever. It's just a matter of fact—a fact that I'm reminded of between one and fifteen times a day. And maybe it's enriching if you take that perspective on it. Maybe I'm afforded a luxury that some people ain't. Maybe I'm afforded a luxury that other people can't purchase. Anybody can buy something to make themselves happy temporarily. But I have something else . . . I'm not in any pain, the people I love and care about ain't in any physical or mental pain. We have some semblance of peace. And that's good enough.

I'll tell you a funny story. I was always a generous type of person—sharp around the edges, sure, but I always try to help people. So, I'm in the cemetery one day, and I'm working with a guy who had lost his daughter to spinal meningitis when she was just five years old. That experience had drawn this man a lot closer to God, and he preached about it all the time. He was a nice guy—a little weird, but a nice guy. One day there's this homeless guy sleeping on the outskirts of the cemetery, up against a fence under some pine trees. And that guy I'd been working with calls the manager and they call the police. Now, I'm twenty or twenty-one at the time, and I was working with a different guy that day. I said to my partner I was working with, "Hey, you got any money on you?" He's like, "Yeah, what's the matter?" I said, "You got, like, twenty bucks? I'll pay you back when I get down to the garage." He gives me forty bucks, "That's all I got." I ran over to the chain-link fence, I slipped the $40 through the fence and I said to the homeless guy, "Hey, you gotta get out of here. The police are coming." And, you know, I'm sitting there thinking: This man, the one who lost his daughter—he's attempting to draw himself closer to God, or to something that can give him peace, because of what he went through, because of this tragedy in his life that I don't know how anyone can recover from. And you have these moments and opportunities to purchase yourself this peace with acts of . . . I dunno, just being a decent fucking person. Black, White, gay, straight, religious, atheist—none of that shit matters, right? None of it really matters if you're just fucking decent to people. I was mind-boggled by this guy (at the time he was like twice my age) who was looking forward to having the cops wrestle this homeless man out. I'm like, "He ain't bothering anybody, man. He's on the outskirts of this thing. Maybe he don't even have peace." It's just weird.

What I'm trying to say is: I think this job's given me that, in certain ways. Sometimes it weighs heavily on you psychologically, emotionally, but in other ways I'm given a little bit of peace. If there's something positive that comes out of all the old-school hard labor and all the shit that I see, it's that it gives me some sort of peace. A good friend of mine said one day, "Hey, man, enjoy things while they're good, because they're definitely not always going to be that way." You know? It's just not always going to be that way. This is temporary; we're all checking out eventually. Maybe we're too smart for our own good, maybe we're too narcissistic. We have this idea of self, this mentality of, "Oh, not me. It won't happen to me." But in reality, it's coming.

Max: Yeah, what do they always say in sports? "Father Time is undefeated."

Nick: Father Time is undefeated. Amen. Amen to that.

Max: Yup.

Nick: But you see what I mean, right? This guy worked with us, and we had come to find out—because he told us—that he was "born again" and all this stuff. And that's great. I didn't subscribe to any type of religious thinking at all at that age, and I don't affiliate with any church or anything now. But what I'm trying to say is: He had this idea of God, religion, worship, and all that, and I believe it was because of his daughter's untimely death. And yet, he had the opportunity to show God, or to live it, or be it, with just a small act of kindness. When you help somebody out like that, you're helping yourself, too. It sounds cliché, but you really are. Whether the homeless guy says, "Thank you," or "Go fuck yourself," you did the right thing as far as I'm concerned. But you just don't kick people when they're down.

That whole thing kind of changed my perspective on this guy. And, look, nobody's perfect—we've all done some bad things. But now I'm sitting there looking at this guy and thinking, "Oh, so you want peace when it's convenient for *you*. You want peace because *you're* hurting. But this homeless guy's hurting; is he not entitled to that peace? He's a human, he lived a life. Maybe he's been through the ringer too, man. Maybe you have more in common with him than you thought." And I'm not like a hippie or nothing. I've definitely clashed with a lot of people before, but I was never somebody to just interact with the intent to hurt somebody, or to see somebody's day become more difficult over stuff like that. As I've gotten older, I went from being a punk kid like, "Hey! What are you lookin' at?" to being like, "You can tell me to go fuck myself, I don't care. As long as you ain't hurting me or the people I care about, we're good."

Max: I think there's really something there, man. Like you said, you're not a hippie or anything, but after seeing the things that you see, after having to go through so much to find that peace you're talking about, the kind of peace money can't buy, there really is a lot of tenderness for humanity, and an understanding of the value and preciousness and temporariness of human life, that I can just hear coming through your stories. Most people don't have that. And who knows? Maybe people are going to come out of all this with a little more of that . . . I don't know. We were just talking about the experience of mass death and what that does to a people and a culture; obviously, we're in the middle of that right now. We've been living through a deadly pandemic over the past year. As we're speaking, I think the official numbers show that over four hundred thousand people in the U.S. have died of COVID-19. Needless to say, it's been a long, arduous, and intense road through this pandemic, and I think most people can't even imagine what it's been like for you and your coworkers. Can we talk about that a bit? Try to put us back in your shoes and see if you can recall what it was like for you—at your job, but also just as a person on this earth, in this country—as the reality of COVID-19 started to set in.

Nick: For me, when COVID hit the news—I guess it was around January of last year—I was like, "Eh." I was a little bit jaded, I guess. I said, "Nah, not here. This is America," you know? "We're exempt from stuff like this, we're unaffected, because we're the greatest country in the world. No dice, not happening here, not on our watch." Then a couple of months went by and it just wasn't going away; people kept talking about it, and it just got bigger and bigger. Every major news channel was talking about it, then they started talking about wearing masks and this and that. I was like, "What? Are you kidding me?" I think what changed it for me—what made "COVID-19" go from just being a name to being something tangible and real—was when I talked to a buddy of mine in the restaurant business. He's been a manager for a chain of restaurants for over twenty-some-odd years—and then, *boom*, very early on, the restaurants went out of business. It happened so fast, like at the drop of a hat. That made me start thinking about the economic impact of the virus.

Then, last year—from, like, April, to May, to June . . . that's something I'll never forget. And it's that experience, in those three months, that makes me question this whole entire COVID thing. I'll elaborate.

Again, there are three cemeteries in my area. At the one where I work, we do an average number of burials daily. The total number of burials we do each year never deviates by more than, like, 50 to 150. At the end of the year, we're always right around the average number, and there's an average number we do on a given day. But in April, May, and June, for three months, we were burying and entombing between ten and fifteen people a day, every day. It was like nothing I've ever experienced in my life. I mean, eight or nine jobs a day: that maybe happens, like, four or five times a year; maybe a dozen at most. But we were doing more than that every day for ninety days. It was crazy. So, I'm thinking to myself, "Wow, everybody's getting infected, and everybody who's getting infected is perishing. This is just nuts!"

But here's the thing, Max: All of a sudden . . . well, not all of a sudden, but at the end of this three-month period . . . we go from ten, twelve, fifteen burials a day to, like, five, six, five, five, four, three, five, three, three, one. It just slid right back to normalcy. So, when the news is covering it now, whether it's a Republican news channel or a Democratic news channel—and, you know, when it comes to covering real things, when it comes to stuff that affects Americans, news should be the same. Unfortunately, with all the politics, it's not . . . but anyway . . . the news is covering it, and they're showing us numbers of deaths and this and that, and I gotta be honest: I'm not experiencing what the media is covering in the cemeteries anymore. Now, are we getting people who died of COVID? Supposedly, yes. What I mean by that is: I'm not denying that they died of COVID. They very well could have, but this is verbal information that directors are communicating to the cemetery: "Hey, just to let you guys know: This person died of COVID." That's what they're saying. Whether they actually died from it, I don't know. Whether it was written on their death certificate, I don't know. I don't want to go too far down that rabbit hole, but my point is that when they talk about this thing spiking and getting really bad again, I don't experience it. It doesn't carry over into the cemeteries. So, I question it . . . I have no choice but to question it.

But I cannot argue with what I experienced for those three months, man. I gotta tell you, just to keep it raw and real: You'd get into work, you'd start at seven-ish, 7:30 a.m., and you'd leave at 5:30 p.m. There were no piss breaks. If you were driving for, like, thirty seconds from one location to the next and you could chug some water in the truck, good for you. If not, you were just S.O.L (Shit Outta Luck). It was insane. We had to put courtesy to the side, cuz we were just running through the cemetery, opening up a hole, putting people in the ground and burying them, putting people in the ground and burying them . . . just no grace whatsoever. And I'm not being dramatic about that. I just can't explain how busy it was. If there's five burials in the location on one day, you're gonna consolidate ten hours' worth of work into an eight-hour day. When there's twelve to fifteen people getting buried, you're consolidating twenty hours of labor into an eight- to ten-hour period.

Max: Jesus. And that's all *on top of* the conditions you already talked about, right? Everything is already so tightly packed and the soil conditions vary so much that you're having to put metal bars in the ground so the remains in neighboring graves don't roll into the hole for the person being buried now. I can only imagine what that was like when you're trying to bury fifteen people in a single day!

Nick: Yeah, there's just a lot of shortcuts, man. I mean, management's not going to write it down and spell it out for you, but they're gonna tell you, "We can't worry about that thing; we just gotta do this, gotta do that." A lot of preventative measures we normally take just went out the window. It was the bare minimum, literally. That translated to cosmetic application: Instead of looking clean and professionally done, it looked like a bomb went off in the area. It also translated to other things. With the water tables, for instance, we usually pump graves with Honda engines and four-inch hoses—that got put to the side. A lot of things got put to the side so that we could, at the very least, provide a resting place *that day* for that individual . . . and for their family.

We were supposedly given government mandates to stay open later so we could accommodate more interments. But the weird thing for me—and maybe I'm just wrong, maybe I'm just ignorant . . . it's very possible . . . What I don't understand is: They talk about how COVID is more contagious and more people are passing, but we're not experiencing that in the cemeteries.

Just to be clear, there's three cemetery locations here in, like, a three-mile perimeter: one's 260 acres, one's 88 acres, one's 48. The 48-acre place is Catholics. The 88-acre place is Chinese, Jewish, and Catholic. And then the other place, the big place, is 90 percent Jewish and probably 10 percent non-sectarian . . . Catholic, Christian, etc. While they're claiming that so many people are passing away from the virus, we're just not seeing that anymore—it's not like it was in the cemetery back in the spring. When it was really bad, and we had these spikes, man, we were crazy for those three months. Now, it's back to normal.

But I know for a fact that it's real. I mean, I got friends and people I know who have gotten the virus: some are asymptomatic, and some still, to this day, are having trouble sleeping. Their bodies won't let them—they've got, like, nerve problems that keep them from falling asleep . . . almost like long haulers, who suffer from that kind of stuff. As for me, I don't think I'm contagious, or I must not be susceptible, because there's no way I can prevent getting COVID from somebody who has it, or from somebody who just died from it. Because, if a person just died from it, and they died last night, and they're getting buried this morning, you're moving that body around, and that body is aspirating that virus; it's all over the place. They're not in a sealed-tight casket, they're not bagged and sealed—none of that is happening. They're in a quarter-inch pine box with wooden dowels—the lid will wobble right off. And then, I gotta go in that grave, and I gotta pull those shale bars out. I gotta hook it up to four-way cables so the backhoe can pull them out. There's so many different, overlapping instances where I would have contracted some sort of viral load of this thing.

Look, maybe I'm just wrong. There's definitely a psychological warfare component, too, right? I see some people masking up in their cars and even in their homes. Me? I do what's mandated out of respect for the person next to me, but I don't live my life in a way that's dominated by this virus, or I try not to. But it's impacted me in other ways, on a personal level: just watching kids—including my own kid—not being able to go to school. But on the job, it's definitely psychological warfare. Because there's days when I say to myself, "I don't even know if this thing exists." And then there's days where I say to myself, "Well, it's got to exist, because the numbers don't lie. Look what happened in April, May, June of 2020." And, again, there's the people I know who got sick, or whose family members got it. It's very up and down.

For me, I'm saying to myself, "This is where I work, this is what it is. If I get it, I get it." I can't prevent it, you know? . . . I can't prevent it. You put a mask on, sure, but you're sweating and sweating—even in the winter, sweating, shoveling, breathing, you gotta touch your face and your hands are full of mud and whatever else. There's just no way. Think about why people wear masks: They wear them so they don't get contact-trace amounts of bacteria or pathogens in their body. Then think about being on a construction site where you're rushing to put people in the ground—just try to remain sanitary in regards to your hands, or mask, or face. I mean, I got lowering devices that weigh eighty-five pounds, I got monuments, four-way cables, center straps, shale bars, brace boards, brace bars, the back-hoe, there's lids, straps, lid cables—there's just so many different things that I'm in contact with. There's no way for me to prevent coming into contact with an aerosolized virus that comes out of people's lungs. And in our place, my company doesn't want to put anything down on paper or say to people, "Due to COVID, we're gonna do this to keep our people safe." For example, at other locations, families aren't even allowed into the cemetery. But us? We take all comers. The governor may put a mandate out that only fifty people are allowed to congregate, but we got three hundred people at the gravesite. So, what we'll do is we'll tell the family, "Hey, stay in your cars, let us lower the casket, and then you can come over and have your service. Then, when you want to see it backfilled, you gotta go back to your vehicles." That's a hard pill to swallow for certain people because they want to be there for all of that. I would say that our policies are extremely lax, especially compared to other places. Is that dangerous? Is that good? Is it bad? I don't know.

Now, look: I'm a person who you could call the victim of something like that, right? If you got two hundred people at a grave, I risk getting infected. But listen: It's their right to see their fucking family get buried. It's somebody else's right to go to a hospital and send their family off or hold their hand. These are things that we, as Americans, are giving up with little resistance out of fear of death. But, like I said earlier, in order to risk living you have to risk dying. It's a hard pill to swallow. I don't think the response to COVID has been run right—obviously, though, it's easy to Monday-morning quarterback and say, "I would do this, I would do that." But I think there are certain things you just don't take away from people, regardless of what the circumstances are. One of those things is being able to hold your loved one's hand as they're dying. Another is putting them to rest in peace at a cemetery. These are basic, primitive things that have been imprinted on us for thousands of years. We raise our people, we take care of them, we feed them, we dote over our young. We bury our dead. These are basic things. And we, as a people, as a society, are just giving that up for this idea of safety.

What's "safe" about something that's exhaled from somebody's lungs into the air? There's nothing safe about that. Now, I'm not saying you should go cough on somebody. We're not talking about going to the store, picking up a cup of coffee, and having to wear a mask. This is bigger than that. This is telling people they can't go to a hospital to see their loved ones because they might get it and bring it home. This is a big deal, and I think it's going to have a profound effect on people. I think the generation coming up is going to be emotionally detached, compared to the people who are going through it now who are emotionally attached. We were talking about the Civil War, right? We were talking about this real, visceral experience that really connected people—these were memories and experiences that were unbreakable, that welded people together. But this? This is like . . . passive crisis. It's like you were saying before: Workers provide the service; a building goes up, but you don't see all that goes into it being built. I think our country is not allowing people to really witness the whole transaction here, whatever that may mean. If it means not visiting somebody in a hospital, or not burying a loved one in accordance with their beliefs or their last will or whatever . . . these are things that we used to call inalienable rights, you know? These weren't rules that were written by men. These were the laws of the land, God's law. These were the ideals America was supposedly founded on. And I think we're all just kind of giving that up. Regardless of who you are, what you are, how you identify politically, and all this other shit, you can't just give that up. But we are, and that's a scary thing.

It's always been the case that you can either have freedom, or you can have safety. The government can provide you with one or the other. But in order to provide you with safety, you have to abide by their demands. And if you hand all your freedom over to the system in exchange for safety, you're not going to get it back. It's like putting gold in somebody's hands and saying, "Hey, hold this for me. I'll come back for it in a few years" . . . not gonna happen. Most people just ain't that honest. Especially people who get into these positions of authority. They don't get there by accident, they don't stumble upon these positions. We've given up a lot of freedom during this pandemic, and we have, in turn, given them a lot more power. I don't know how this is all gonna shake out, I don't know what they're gonna do with that power, but I think COVID is gonna usher in a new kind of system, and it's gonna change the world. I really do . . . I really do.

2. Rebecca Garelli

My name is Rebecca Garelli. I am a science and STEM specialist in Arizona, and I work full-time organizing educators. I'm a lead organizer with Arizona Educators United, which is really the "Red for Ed" movement down here in Arizona, and with National Educators United. I'm thirty-nine, and I'm a mom of three kids under the age of seven.

Max: There's so much I want to talk to you about, Rebecca. But honestly, I wanted to start by just asking: How are you doing? How are you and your family holding up during all of this?

Rebecca: Every day feels like Groundhog Day, quite frankly: I get up, I do the same thing. My children are all remote learning currently, which means that our schedules are intense and a little bit crazy. I'm fortunate enough to be safe and working from home. Since the schools have closed, my husband had to voluntarily quit his job and is on unemployment now so he can stay home and take care of our kids. And so . . . I think we're okay. It's really challenging with three little kids who don't have playdates, don't have soccer, they don't have their friends at school, or recess, or the things that normalize their lives. But in light of all of that, we are healthy and we're safe. We spend most of our time just making sure our kids are as happy as can be, getting outdoors as much as possible and doing some hiking. We've been relying on the beautiful weather of Arizona to help us through this. But really, it's Groundhog Day . . . and it's exhausting.

On the organizing side of things: It's demoralizing, intensely demoralizing, to witness what's happening here in Arizona. Educators are being pushed back into in-person learning in very, very unsafe conditions without mitigation efforts, without testing at schools. It's really demoralizing, that's the best word I can come up with to describe it. As an organizer, you understand demoralization; you understand that it's hard to organize folks, and even harder to organize in digital spaces during a pandemic.

Mentally, it's really a struggle to want to do what's right for your children and your family but finances are really tight. We're really struggling with it, because unemployment in Arizona is the lowest in the nation; it doesn't come close to the income level that my husband used to bring in. Between finances and depression with our kids, to hoping we can get through, to organizing educators . . . it's a lot. But we're really trying to be grateful for what we have in our own space, and we're trying to keep our kids healthy and safe at the same time.

Max: I want to ask you a little more about this, because this is something that I think we're all dealing with in some capacity: the immense emotional and psychological toll that living through the COVID-19 pandemic has taken on all of us. As you said, even for those of us who have been fortunate enough to be able to work from home, or to at least be able to survive at home, it has still been rough. It puts so much pressure on our psyches to be living in isolation like this, to be so cut off from the human touches and connections that we have always been able to take for granted. Personally, going through this has just made me realize, more and more, how much I need people, how much we all need one another. That social life, that being-together, is such an essential part of living on this earth that if you *don't* have those in-person connections to your fellow human beings, you literally start wasting away. You lose so much of what you call yourself when you're living in these conditions. I know I do: I can't sleep as well; I get depressed; I find it much harder to get myself out of those periods of depression. This whole experience has shown me that, to be a functioning human being in this world, I need other people.

But, of course, this pandemic has also had really intense consequences for people who haven't had the ability to stay at home, people who have had to risk their lives and their health by going outside and working, because they wouldn't have the support they need to pay rent or buy groceries otherwise. Like you said, this is a really important and serious issue for educators, who are currently being forced back to in-person learning while the death and infection rates are still sky high. You've got a lot of school districts, mayors, and state houses all saying the same thing: "We need to force students, teachers, and staff back to in-person learning, because it's too damaging to students' long-term development to keep them learning remotely for so long." That's the argument they're using to justify pushing everyone back into schools before it's safe.

Now, you are kind of straddling a number of these difficult realities at once: as a parent with your own children, as someone who has been an educator herself and who works to organize educators now. Could you talk a little more about how you, and others you've talked to, have been trying to navigate all of this?

Rebecca: When it comes to that specific argument about the mental health and well-being of students, educators already know this. We have been charged with the responsibility of being mental health specialists on top of our normal professional duties, which is wrong to begin with. Here in the U.S., even before the pandemic started, this is a job that was basically plopped in our laps: "You're now going to be the mental health worker in your space with these students, because, due to funding, we don't have counselors in every single building." Now, I've been an educator for seventeen years. I spent most of my career, thirteen years, as a middle school math and science educator, as well as a few years as a science instructional coach and adjunct faculty at DePaul University STEM Center. Before I got to Arizona, I was in the Chicago Teachers Union, so I've been paying attention for quite a while. And I can tell you: This is a false narrative. It's ridiculous. If people *really* cared about students' mental health, especially the decision makers who are using this narrative to force people back to school, you would have funded counselors in every single building, and you haven't. In Arizona, the student-to-counselor ratio is 903-1. On my campus (I taught in West Phoenix), we had one counselor for 1,900 students; we shared one counselor between two campuses. Even when I was teaching in Chicago, we didn't have a counselor every day; maybe it would be on Tuesdays, or Tuesdays and Thursdays. When there was a student crisis and I'd pick up the phone and try to call for a counselor to come in and intervene or help . . . it wasn't there. If we actually cared about our students' mental health, we would be giving full funding for counselors to be in every single school across the nation, five days a week.

This isn't to say the concerns aren't real, though. I see the toll this is all taking on the mental health of my own kids. We have days where we go through sadness; we're missing our friends and don't understand why we can't see our friends. So, I'm not saying mental health isn't a concern of all educators; obviously, it is. We *care* about our kids. To say we don't is unbelievably untrue.

And then to navigate the pandemic as a mom, it's about finding a balance, right? It's about helping my kids, who are very young and were just starting to make friends at school. I have a six-year-old and four-year-old twins. It's really hard for them, they don't understand why we can't go home to Chicago, why we haven't seen our family there in over a year. "Why can't we go see Nana? Why can't we see our friends? Why can't we do our soccer league?" So, as a mom, I understand the mental health issue very intimately, but as a teacher, I think using that as a reason to force people back into unsafe working conditions is really quite disgusting.

Max: I think you hit the nail on the head. If this was *really* the thing these people cared about, then there are, like, ten other steps they could have taken before we arrived at, "We need everyone to go back to in-person learning!" It's such bullshit, man.

Rebecca: Totally.

Max: This whole thing has just got me thinking . . . I'm not a parent, I can't speak to that experience. But as we've been living through this pandemic, and as we've been hearing so many of these arguments from public officials and pundits about the mental health of schoolchildren, I can't help but try to think about what I would have done if I was a kid going through something like this. You and I grew up at a time when, thankfully, we never had to go into quarantine for a year. As a parent, it must be so scary to try to help your children navigate this when you yourself never experienced anything like that when you were growing up. Has that been playing on your mind? When you put the kids to bed and you're up at night thinking, have you ever wondered what we would have done if we had to go through something like this when we were their age?

Rebecca: Yes, but more in a superficial sort of way. It'll be like, "Man, we are really fortunate to live in Arizona where the weather's nice and we can all jump in the pool." I grew up in Chicago: We understood what Seasonal Affective Disorder was growing up . . .

Max: [Laughs.]

Rebecca: Honestly, just having that sun out every single day and being able to go outside during the winter is one of the biggest things supporting what we do here in this family. I haven't necessarily been thinking of what we would do as kids. More than anything, I've just been grateful for what we have now. It's like, "Man, I'm really happy we have iPad games for every single kid, how fortunate are we?" We struggled to find the money for iPads, but we were finally able to scrounge up some cash, and we needed them, because, just from a basic, material standpoint, it was really challenging for teachers to build lessons and support our kids without them. It's already hard enough, and it takes a physical and mental toll, to plan lessons and get your kids to do the work. Doing that remotely is a whole other animal.

To answer your question, I don't think I've ever really sat down to think, "If this were happening back in the '80s or '90s when I was growing up, what would we be doing?" I guess we would have played a lot of Monopoly or Nintendo? It's more like, "Man, I'm really grateful we have X and Y." And my mom has been supporting us by sending us glue, construction paper, art supplies, and other things to help with our kids' growth and development; nurturing that creative aspect of my children's brains at this crucial time in their lives is so important. More than anything, I just feel really lucky that we have all these things to help us be safe and healthy and mentally capable, things that help improve my kids' educational opportunities here at home. We have the tools to help us survive in the best way possible now, we're fortunate enough to have the ability to do remote learning in virtual classrooms.

Max: And I know that this is a really important issue when it comes to the work that you've been doing, not only as an educator but as an organizer, right? Those tools you're talking about have also made it more possible to do the work of organizing, even during a deadly pandemic. I wanted to ask if you could talk a bit about that: What have those same technologies allowed you to do as a full-time organizer? And what sorts of obstacles has the pandemic posed for your organizing work?

Rebecca: I love this question. As organizers, this is something we reflect upon quite often. What these tools have allowed us to do is get a lot of people in a space. Organizing is about opening spaces; it's about listening to people and figuring out which issues are widely and deeply felt. The way we organize here in Arizona is statewide: We have built an external structure beyond the actual union structures, and we've done that using the Facebook group "Arizona Educators United." That's been kind of a powerhouse Facebook group since the 2018 strike[1] and we've continued to use it as one of our main vehicles for organizing, and we're linked to, like, sixty-five other Facebook pages connecting us to different districts across the state. If we need a message to get out, or if we need to promote an event, or if we want to support educators in a certain district, we have these vehicles and structures for doing so that we had built back in 2018 and that we can activate now. Even before the pandemic, the nature of our organizing was initially online, so we've benefited from that over the past year.

Obviously, though, we also face the obstacle of getting people into in-person spaces. We used to be able to meet people in large spaces; we'd get a union hall, or we'd meet at a coffee shop or someone's house. But now that everybody's more comfortable in a Zoom setting . . . or Webex, or Google Meet, or whatever . . . we're able to use Zoom meetings quite frequently to organize folks and get people into a space. And now, with these tools we're using—we've got breakout rooms and strategies for digital organizing meetings, we've got digital tools for coming to a consensus vote, and

---

1 From April 26 to May 3, 2018, 20,000 teachers across the state of Arizona went on strike to protest years of austerity measures gutting funding for education and pay rates for teachers and staff. After rejecting a proposal from Arizona Governor Doug Ducey that would have raised teachers' pay by 20 percent by 2020 but provided no additional funding for schools or raises for support staff, the strike successfully secured more concessions from the state government, including salary increases for school staff and reduced student-to-counselor ratios. The Arizona strike occurred within a "wave" of educator-led strikes during 2018–2019 in states like West Virginia, Oklahoma, Colorado, and California known as the "Red for Ed" movement.

there are education tools we use in the classroom, like a jam board, or Padlet, or a Whiteboard—we're helping teachers learn how to organize their students. I don't necessarily mean "organize" in a "Fight back!" kind of way. It's more like: We implement digital tools in our meetings and teachers go, "Oh, I could use that with my students in social studies or math." And we go, "Yeah! Here's a strategy for group voting. Here's a strategy for coming to consensus. Here's a strategy to get everybody's ideas on paper and to move the work forward."

I build science webinars for a living. I teach teachers science, and I teach them how to best use digital tools in the classroom. Now I have a new space as an organizer to help people find these same tools; that's amazing. And they have also helped us in other respects. We have to put out a lot of fires here, you know? There's a lot of "this district versus that district" stuff, because our governor chose to divide and conquer, putting the onus on individual districts to make the life-and-death decisions about when to reopen schools. And, frankly, they're failing miserably in some districts. They're just being complete bad actors. So, we've been able to target different districts, get people from those districts, bring them into a space, and say, "How can we support you? What's going on over there? What's your union doing? Do we need to do something outside of the union?" We can just walk them through the organizing process, step by step. They might want to write a petition, so we'll say, "Alright, before you write a petition, let's go back: You got to get people into a space, you got to start contacting people, we got to find issues that are widely and deeply felt."

We have ways to connect to people all across the state, which might have been trickier if people weren't so comfortable in the online space. One of the biggest obstacles, though, is getting to the parents. Parent organizing is very tricky, especially because the ones you want to connect with and organize are the ones whose kids are remote: Even if you came up with an informational picket, or a walk-in, or some other action that you could do visibly at the school, you're really only going to be meeting the opposition, the parents who are demanding their kids go to school in person, the loudest ones, the ones who don't listen to science. It's really sad to say they're the opposition, but they are. They're the ones you see at the schools, they're the ones dropping their kids off.

Max: This raises a question that has always really fascinated me, because we're touching on something that anyone invested in the labor movement writ large thinks about a lot, or knows very intimately, right? This is something that organizers like yourself are doing on a daily basis: You talk to people, you identify people's strengths and skills, and you find ways to harness those skills for the collective benefit of the movement. That's such important work. I remember talking to a woman in New Orleans who works as a waitress by day and an organizer by night, and she said something I'll never forget. She said service workers make some of the best organizers. For instance, we talked about the fact that she and her coworkers have to code switch all the time as part of their job, because so many different types of customers are entering the coffee shop at different points in their day, their needs and attitudes vary so much depending on the different circumstances of their lives, and, as a customer-service employee, you have to constantly navigate and adjust to that. Being able to do that is a skill, and there's obviously a tremendous amount of value in being able to take those skills and apply them in a political context. It takes all of us to build a movement, and we all have so many skills to bring to that movement.

Rebecca: Definitely.

Max: I wanted to talk a little about that, specifically in relation to you as an educator and an organizer. Just hearing the way you talk about this stuff, it's very clear that you think a lot about harnessing and transferring these kinds of skills. Clearly there are many things you've learned through your work with Educators United that you have translated into something educators can use in the classroom, but it also sounds like there are things you learned in the classroom that you have brought into your organizing. So, there's kind of a chicken and egg question there, right? [Laughs.] Do you think that being a natural-born organizer made you a better teacher? Or did being a natural-born teacher make you a better organizer?

Rebecca: I absolutely love this question, because I've been trying to sell people on the idea that educators *are* the best organizers. I think about this all the time. We are the best teachers, we know how to plan, we know how to get someone from A to B. When I think about how I got here, and how my brain functions as an organizer, it's all connected to the things I do well as an educator: I'm a planner, I lay things out, I think about outcomes and what to do with them . . . "What am I going to do to move from outcome A to outcome B? If I get a different outcome, what does that tell me? And how can I work out a different path to achieve a different outcome?"

I don't know about the chicken or the egg; I just know that my brain has always functioned this way. Back in high school, I was a pretty talented athlete, especially in basketball. My mom and I used to talk about this all the time. She would say, "You can just see the floor and all the moving parts, and you just know instinctively how to get the ball where it needs to be." And she was right, my brain just makes those connections like bing-bing-bing-bing, A to B, B to C.

That translated into being really good at math and science my whole life, and being able to solve a problem using mathematics, engineering, or something along those lines. When I translated that into teaching, I think it just allowed me to become better at the things I was already naturally good at. I've always been really good at planning things and thinking sequentially and logically about first steps, second steps, third steps. I'm a linear thinker: I have a way of looking at things, putting them in a certain order to achieve a specific outcome, etc. And that's teaching, really.

I started teaching basketball way back in the day when I was, like, eighteen. When I was in college, I worked for a company called One on One Basketball, and that was really how I got into teaching. I would teach after-school basketball programs, summer camps, clinics . . . this was all in Chicago . . . and I got to learn the public school system and the private school system, because I was invested in coming into those buildings and working with the kids. Eventually I realized, "I'm really good at explaining basketball to people. Maybe I'm really good at being a teacher. Maybe that's just a thing I'm naturally good at." That's how I got into teaching in the first place. Teaching kids how to be really good at basketball, being able to explicitly explain something to them, then having them take that knowledge and achieve a positive outcome with it: I really enjoyed that.

Again, I don't know about the chicken or the egg question; I just know that, on a weekly basis, I think about how educators make the best organizers *because* of these skills we develop. This is literally what we do on a daily basis: We have to plan, and we have to switch if the plan isn't working out. "Okay, this thing isn't working, I'm gonna adjust. I'm gonna figure out a different way to approach X and see if the kids will come with me." You've got to do the same thing with organizing: The minute you get stuck down one path, you have to stop and say, "Well, I'm not going to keep forcing it, because that's not going to work. This isn't giving me the outcome that I want." Just like with teaching, you have to step back and say, "What might work instead?" Maybe that's part of the "code switching" you're talking about. Here we talk more about "sugarcoating" or, you know, not speaking as militantly in mixed company as we would in our own spaces. Because it's about messaging, it's about bringing people in, finding their comfort zone, and meeting them where they're at; that's the only way you're going to move them forward. And that's what teaching is, that's what teachers do. Whether you're teaching math, science, or whatever, the minute you get a new group of kids, you figure out where they're at, then you figure out a plan to help move them forward.

Max: I can't help myself, but since you brought up basketball . . .

Rebecca: [Laughs.]

Max: I played basketball my whole life, from elementary school through varsity in high school, and I played pickup like three to four times a week during college and after. I *loved* playing basketball, right up until the moment I blew out my knee playing one-on-one in grad school—tore my ACL, MCL, and meniscus. I haven't been able to play since . . . not like I could before, at least . . . and I really mourn the loss of the role basketball played in my life and the joy that it brought me.

Anyway, I bring it up because I think it's such a great analogy, and there's really something to take to heart in what you were saying. It makes me think of this debate I've had with so many people over the years: Someone always wants to argue that sports, especially in this country, have no political value. But the conversation is usually limited to professional sports, and they only talk about sports as an entertainment product, a spectacle to consume. People think they're being smart when they say stuff like, "The Super Bowl is just a gross capitalist and nationalist spectacle!" Yeah, no shit! But these sorts of conversations rarely focus on the experience of playing sports yourself, the necessity of involving yourself in that act of play, and what that experience can mean for you as a developing human being.

Because, like you were saying, if you're playing basketball, you are working with a finite group of people on a finite court with boundaries and rules, and it's within that kind of environment that you are able to *create*, to push yourself and your teammates to accomplish things you didn't even know you were capable of. That's why this is such a hard thing to communicate to anyone who doesn't play sports, because we don't really have many other areas of our social existence where we can experience the kind of creativity, play, and teamwork we experience playing sports. There just aren't many other experiences to compare it to. That's also why sports are *very* politically valuable, along with being fun and joyful and good for our health. If you're playing a game of pickup basketball, you're a member of a team, right? You have to strategize, you have to identify quickly what your team's strengths and weaknesses are, and you gotta try to make those strengths complement each other and work together to achieve a common goal. These are politically impor-tant skills, too, and they require practice. There's so much that you learn through the experience of playing that has value on and off the court, just like, as you said, there's so much you learn through the experience of being an educator that has tremendous value within and beyond the classroom.

We don't have to go farther down that rabbit hole [laughs], but let me use this as a chance to reframe the chicken and egg question and ask, instead: From your experience playing sports to your experience in the classroom, what do you think really laid the path for you to become a professional organizer?

Rebecca: This is not the first time I've been asked this question. It's always fun to think back and reflect on the path that led me here. I do think sports helped me understand power in my personal life, and there was something very valuable in that. Sports gave me my first taste of what it felt like to feel powerful. Because I was very good at three sports, I played varsity in three sports for all of high school, I became the captain of the team, and I understood that my voice mattered. When I spoke, people listened. Being an awkward high-schooler, that was my first taste of feeling like, "Oh, I guess I *am* a leader. Okay." The identification and acknowledgement that I do have leadership skills was something that I never truly internalized until I became a team leader on the basketball court, the softball field, or whatever. I think that is how, little by little, I came to understand power within myself. I was always a really silent kind of kid; I was a good student, but just pretty quiet. My mom had always referred to me as a "silent leader." She jokes about that a lot. She'll say, "You used to be a silent leader, but you're not silent anymore."

Thinking about my path to becoming an organizer, it really did start with that silent leader kind of mentality: I shut up and did my work. I had my own thoughts that were sometimes very different from what other people thought, but I kept quiet. But when I got on the basketball court people looked to me to save the day. I was the guy who made the game-winning shot or whatever. And then the power of teaching kids how to become good at basketball gave me my second inkling of feeling like, "Wow, I'm really making a difference here. These kids love this, I love this. This is great!"

Then I became a teacher. Now, when you become a teacher, everyone has these tipping points, and I'll tell you about mine. I went to DePaul University in Chicago, and I went into a pretty progressive program. The title of the program is not my favorite; it was called the "Multicultural/Urban Educator Program." The point, really, was to immerse us within Chicago Public Schools. I got to work in my own community, I could walk to the school, and the kids all lived around me. I had started teaching in Chicago in 2004, and throughout the course of my undergrad work I was immersed in a lot of different Chicago Public Schools and different communities.

After I graduated, though, I had a really hard time finding a job; there weren't a lot of jobs in Chicago and I basically had to take what I could get. I ended up subbing for a year at one school on the North Side called Ravenswood. Then I got a job on the West Side and, man . . . that was a tipping point for me. I remember I had spent the entire Labor Day weekend getting everything ready; I probably spent, I dunno, $250 getting all this new, fun stuff for the kids, decorating the classroom, etc. I was really pumped about it. Then I show up on the first day of school and the principal brings me into the office and says, "I'm really sorry to tell you this, but I don't have a position for you." And I was like, "Excuse me?" Basically, what happened is she had lied to me and put me under the wrong bucket number coding. A bucket number is a line item in a school's budget. Certain bucket numbers are designated for educators with specific credentials, like a music or art teacher, a school nurse, special education, and general-education-certificate educators. When interviewed, I was offered the position for a seventh grade science teaching position, which matches my credentials and certifications. However, to maneuver around some budget line items, the principal placed me in a bucket number as a music teacher, and I am *certainly* not a music teacher. No music credentials whatsoever. And I thought, "This is insane."

Max: [Laughs.]

Rebecca: This budgetary maneuver ended up causing me to lose my position since I had no seniority, no tenure, and was a new hire. The way school funding works is that it is based on enrollment; the principal made enrollment projections and budget decisions, including decisions about the number of staff positions, based on projections. Well, it turned out that actual student enrollment at the beginning of the year was much lower than projected, which, simply put, means loss of teaching positions, including mine. So, I had to literally pack up everything from my classroom and put it all into my car right then and there. I called my mom and she told me, "Call the union. Call H.R." So I did. I called H.R. and said to them, "You need to find me a position, stat. This is what happened, this is wrong. If you don't want me to take any more action, you're gonna find me a job right now." And they did. After that, I went back into the principal's office and said, "You owe me three days' worth of pay, and I'm not going to stop until you pay me for those days." And she basically wrote me a personal check for $700. To me, that was one more taste of power. A lot of people probably would have just shut up and gone on their way, especially if they're non-tenured teachers. But I didn't. I knew it was wrong, and I knew I had to say something. So, I did.

After I called H.R. at Chicago Public Schools, they put me in a substitute position that was walking distance from my house. I worked and lived in the Wicker Park/Ukrainian Village area. *That* is the school where I learned about union power. Somehow, I feel like I was destined to be there. Teaching there was my big tipping point; it's why I'm an organizer today. After the horrible mess at the other school, I came to this school, where I was supposed to fill in teaching first grade for a lady who was on medical leave. She needed someone for, like, half a year, and I was happy to do it. Now, the principal at the time was one of those guys who just really wanted to climb the ladder, only had five years of experience in the classroom, not on the side of educators at all. Basically, he paid me as a substitute when I should have been paid as a regular Temporary Assigned Teacher (TAT).

I remember I kept looking at my paychecks and thinking, "Something's wrong." So, I called my mom again (cuz my mom's amazing) and was like, "Mom, what do I do?" She said, "Rebecca, go to the union," so I went to the union. Thankfully, I had the most incredible union rep in my building named Stephanie Collins. She's retired now, but still organizing as the co-chair of the Black Caucus for the Chicago Teachers Union. I am beyond grateful for her. She is the reason I'm here. So, I said to Stephanie, "Here's what's happening. I think something's wrong with my paycheck and I'm getting paid as a substitute, not as a certified teacher."

Stephanie goes, "Alright, here's what we're gonna do. You're gonna meet me outside the office and we're gonna talk and we're gonna say the word 'grievance' out loud." I was like, "Okay, I'm down. Let's do this." And so, we met outside the office, we brought the paperwork to file a grievance, and Stephanie brought with her the other veteran teachers to meet me. We met publicly, we said the words out loud so that people could overhear. We just kind of played this game a little bit, because filing a grievance against a principal is very bad; they don't want that to happen. But it's power. I learned right there and then that even the word "grievance" is power.

We kept having these meetings on Fridays. The principal would see me with all these veteran teachers—he knew what we were up to. It was really the union saying, "We'll go with you, we'll help you fight this." And, sure enough, the principal figured out how to get me my backpay and my rights; he figured out how to get me on the right bucket number and make sure that I was paid what I was supposed to be paid. It was so disgusting, though, because I was gonna get about $10,000, and I remember he looked right at me and said, "Well, aren't you glad? I acted like your savings account!" Right there, right then, I was like, "You are the enemy. You are management, you are the boss. I am now a union thug."

That was the most disgusting treatment I had ever experienced in my life—or one of the most disgusting instances, at least. I learned quickly that if I hadn't gone to the union, I wouldn't be here. They fought for me, and they fixed it in, like, less than two months. I had this guy on my back, and I wasn't a tenured teacher yet, but I learned to stand tall. Eventually, I became an advocate in my building, and I got elected to the local school council a couple years later—that was around 2007. Then, in 2012, we went on strike in Chicago.[2] And so, all

2 In September 2012, around 26,000 members of the Chicago Teachers Union (CTU) went on strike. The strike, which lasted seven school days, was the union's first since 1987—a quarter of a century. At a time when organized labor writ large was taking beatings and accepting concessions left and right—a trend that was accelerated during the Great Recession—CTU was revamping its union philosophy and rebuilding its organizing strategy around a more democratic, militant, and progressive model of social justice unionism. Having voted in a new slate of leaders from the Caucus of Rank and File Educators (CORE) in 2010, the union focused on mobilizing its rank-and-file members and connecting the workplace struggles of educators to the needs and concerns of students, parents, and their communities. These efforts would prove vital for the union's successes during the strike as it went up against the powerfully allied forces of Chicago mayor Rahm Emanuel, the Chicago Public Schools (CPS) administration and Board of Education, and a slew of wealthy, pro-charter school, anti-union actors and private foundations. As Steven Ashby and Robert Bruno note in their seminal book on the CTU strike, *A Fight for the Soul of Public Education: The Story of the Chicago Teachers Strike*, "For many years prior to the events in Chicago, Illinois politicians and business leaders had pushed education reforms that blamed teachers for all the problems in Chicago's schools, sought to break the ability of teachers unions to negotiate over classroom issues, and prioritized the systematic closing of public schools and their replacement with privately run but publicly funded and often for-profit charter schools . . . Where past union leaders had largely ignored the CPS administration's and the mayor's trampling on teacher professionalism, and union leaders had disavowed membership mobilization to counter corporate reform measures, the CORE activists seemed fearless in their willingness to educate, organize, and mobilize CTU members and their allies to resist." While the strike ended with both sides making concessions, the very fact that CTU was able to wage such a strong, unified, and community-allied fight was an inspiration to many unions and workers around the country and beyond, and many labor scholars point to the 2012 CTU strike as a critical turning point in the U.S. labor movement that would provide a model for increased organizing efforts and strikes in the ensuing decade. The task of trying to condense the history and importance of such a pivotal strike into a footnote is absurd and impossible, so I would highly recommend reading Ashby and Bruno's book to learn more, as well as: *Worth Striking For: Why Education Policy Is Every Teacher's Concern (Lessons from Chicago)* by Isabel Nuñez, Gregory Michie, and Pamela Konkol; *How to Jump-Start Your Union* by Labor Notes; *Strike for America: Chicago*

of these things helped put me on this path to being an advocate and an organizer. They helped me say, "This is wrong, and I'm going to do something about it. I'm not going to apologize and I'm not going to be afraid." In retrospect, that is literally how I have acted my whole life. I just don't stand down. When there's injustice, I speak up. The difference was: Now that I had a union, I felt what it was like to have the power to do something about it.

That's kind of my journey here. Getting that union mentality in Chicago, having a union say, "We got your back, no matter what"—that just stuck with me forever. And that has really helped me in Arizona, because when I came out here, I was like, "My gosh, what are these working conditions? This is horrific!" So, yeah, I learned about power pretty early on in my career—and I had a strong personality to begin with, so that helped. I'm not somebody who shies away from conflict: It doesn't make me feel awkward. I find power in resolving conflict. It makes me feel good, and I'm not afraid to do it.

Max: That's so awesome. The educators you work with and represent are so lucky to have you. And this is all really relevant and important, because I imagine anyone reading this has at least had this kind of experience at some point in their life: having a boss fuck you over, not getting the pay you deserve, having no one to turn to, not having any representation or coworkers who have your back. It's a really scary and isolating experience to have someone with that much power over you and to feel so powerless against it. Experiencing that powerlessness is practically a rite of passage for working people.

Think about all those so-called "starter jobs" you get right out of high school. You go and work in fast food, retail, etc., and it almost feels like the purpose of pushing so many people into these largely low-wage, non-union jobs is to educate us in the experience of powerlessness—to acculturate us to being part of a workforce in which we have no one else to turn to. We're taught to expect that our managers and bosses are going to have this largely unchecked power to dictate how we live

Teachers Against Austerity by Micah Uetricht; and A Political Education: Black Politics and Education Reform in Chicago since the 1960s by Elizabeth Todd-Breland.

our lives. And then we're taught to take that same kind of acceptance—acceptance of fundamental class hierarchies that appear permanent and unquestionable, acceptance of top-down authority from people who are not really bound by the same rules we are—and apply it to practically every other aspect of our lives and the world around us. It's a really weird and cruel form of social engineering, I think. But, like you were saying, the opposite is also true: If you do have that experience of being empowered in the workplace, of feeling supported by a union, or (if you don't have a union) of just feeling solidarity with your coworkers, that's equally impactful.

Rebecca: Absolutely. And winning! When you think about power and the struggle for power, experiencing a win is the most incredible feeling in the world. Taking action and following through until you win—that's what it's all about, right?

Max: Oh, definitely. That's a really powerful, formative experience for people who live in a society that works every day to convince us that we're powerless. I suppose that brings me to another question, which is about the work that you've been doing during the pandemic and the obstacles you and other educators have faced.

You mentioned the Chicago teachers' strike of 2012, the Arizona educators' strike in 2018, and you brought up the fact that, long before the pandemic hit our shores, there were *a lot* of problems with the public education system in the United States. In a way, a terrible event like COVID-19 has shown us all just how ill-prepared our system is to handle anything like this, because it has been deliberately and methodically gutted, hollowed out, and because worker protections have been stripped over decades. So much of our public infrastructure and social safety net has been destroyed that we . . . that is, non-rich people . . . really entered this pandemic at a severe disadvantage. At our hour of need, when essential services were more essential than ever, the system buckled . . . it failed us. How have these pre-existing problems shaped the terrain that you and the folks you work with are on? How have you been able to bring that fighting spirit and focus on building power when you're not only combatting a pandemic but a rotted public system?

Rebecca: I think by January of 2020 we had all heard about COVID, and there was a lot of waiting and whispering about when it would enter the United States. All the while, though, everybody in educator spaces, whether online or in actual meetings—we all knew what was coming. It was clear as day that all the injustices of our education system—lack of funding, massive class sizes, lack of teachers, lack of substitutes, lack of counselors—all that lacking was gonna come to light. COVID just exposed everything we already knew about the state of public education across the nation. It just amplified these problems tenfold and put them on display. A lot of people who really might not have understood what happens in the classroom, what we deal with on a daily basis—they might have a better idea now.

As educators, we know that what we do is the cornerstone of democracy, we know that the economy relies entirely upon our labor and the variety of services we provide—specifically, childcare. We know all of these things. We also knew that the minute COVID got here we were all going to be subjected to austerity conversations, because we're used to having our budgets slashed. We're used to people saying, "No, you can't have X, Y, or Z," and we knew it was going to be the same thing when it came to securing PPE and implementing basic sanitation measures. As educators and organizers, we knew that we were going to experience budget cuts, and we knew we were going to have to bear the brunt of society, like we always do. With all the concern around the country right now for students' mental health, everybody else in the nation is getting a little taste of what educators deal with every day. To be honest, at the beginning of the pandemic, we thought there could be positive side effects to that. We thought, "Oh, now that schools are shut down and students are learning remotely, parents are really going to see what we do." And for a short time around March and April, there was this sympathetic sentiment toward educators and the dignified work we do; more people realized how hard this work is, and we were happy about that. It was like, "Hey, people are looking at us in this new light. We're not the enemy anymore. This is great." But it lasted for, like, two seconds.

Here in Arizona, school years end in the third week of May. So, we stayed in remote learning through the end of the year, then we had the summer. Over the summer, though, we were all thinking, "Oh, my goodness. What metrics are they going to use to bring us back to in-person learning? Who is going to be making these decisions? And how are we going to know what science is informing those decisions?" I mean, our minds just exploded over the summer, quite frankly. Come June, I think I was in about four hours of organizing meetings every single day. It was really challenging to try to figure out the playbook for how to proceed, because we've never been through something like this; we could try to guess and speculate and say, "Well, we think X is going to happen, so how do we prepare for that with a campaign? How do we organize ourselves for the fights that are on the horizon?"

I ended up joining in coalition with teacher unionists across the nation: folks with United Teachers of L.A., the Chicago Teachers Union, folks in West Virginia and Baltimore—all the progressive unions. We formed the Demand Safe Schools Coalition with community partners like Journey for Justice and The Center for Popular Democracy. We had been having conversations since March about, "What things are we all seeing? How can we work together? What are the right demands?" It was just so intense and so insane. Across the nation, people were talking about all the things impacting our students, but not the responsibilities that all of this put on teachers. But that also means we've been put in a very crucial position.

Again, we are basically the keepers of the economy, right? Without us, the economy doesn't function. Over the summer, we were thinking, "We're at the vanguard of the labor movement right now. We have complete power in this instance—if we're organized." And so, we had to think about what was going to happen in all of our different spaces across the nation, and about how we could unite to fight back, nationally and locally, with a clear message. Come July, we were protesting at the Capitol. We had car caravans, and our messaging was clear: "We will not go back until it's safe." Then, month after month, we just watched the system work the way it was designed to work and do what it was designed to do: divide us, pit us against each other. The division is just mind-blowing: worker versus worker, bus drivers versus classified staff, parents versus educators.

As far as the organizing we've been doing this entire time, both locally and nationally, we've focused on a number of issues. Education, for one. We brought in industrial hygienists to educate folks about ventilation and to help us understand the aerosolized nature of these particles. They showed us that staying six feet apart isn't good enough, because those particles can travel up to twenty-six feet. And, I mean, we have a lot of windows in classrooms that don't open, so they showed us that proper ventilation means, "You need this kind of filter. If you can't get this kind of filter, you need to get this kind of HEPA [high-efficiency particulate absorbing] filtration unit for your classroom." As a science educator, this was my kind of thing, and educating people about the science—"What are the myths? What are the facts?"—was an extremely important focus of our efforts. But it was also very tricky, and it's still tricky. Because there *are* districts doing the right thing. Our urban progressive districts—the ones serving predominantly disadvantaged communities, Black and Brown communities—have done the right thing. They said loud and clear, "This virus is disproportionately affecting our communities. We're not opening; we're not doing it." However, in other districts, like in the suburbs of Phoenix (where I'm at), you have these anti-masker, anti-science people demanding in-person learning, people with a very my-tax-dollars-pay-your-salary kind of mentality. It's disgusting.

We had such power in 2018. We organized statewide. We organized over 1,200 schools and had over 2,000 volunteer liaisons. A liaison functions as a union site rep or steward for each individual school, and we had two thousand of them! The liaison's role was to serve as an intermediary between the main organizing team of Arizona Educators United and the rank and file at the school site. We asked folks to step up and join the movement as a liaison, and they did. We continually provided organizing strategies and gave them instructions on how to organize their workplace. For example, we asked them to complete actions, map their workplace to identify new leaders and allies, and provide feedback to our core organizing team throughout the eight weeks of organizing. They served as rank-and-file workplace leaders; they were the "boots on the ground," so to speak. This liaison role was vital to the movement—it's what helped us build our massive, statewide network, and build our collective power.

We were united then, but it's hard to be united right now. We are certainly trying to build that solidarity and stress to people that, you know, "All of our communities are interconnected. Whether you're remote or not, we all need to do this together; otherwise, our communities aren't safe." Sadly, what's happening in Arizona is proving that point. Right now, in January 2021, we are number one in the world in terms of COVID positivity per capita. This is the third time during the pandemic that Arizona has made that chart. The blatant disregard for human life is just staggering, and our government is currently trying to vaccinate its way out of this mess. Yes, it's good that teachers are getting vaccinated here, and I know in other places around the country that's not the case.

But we've already lost eleven thousand Arizonans. So, from an organizing perspective, the unity just isn't there as much as it should be. In 2018 funding was the issue that unified us. Everybody—Republicans, Democrats, Independents—could unite in agreement that public schools were underfunded. Now, finding that kind of unity is tricky because we have districts that are doing things safely and we have districts that are not. And, more than anything, people are just exhausted. Even if they understand what we're telling them, even if they understand that our communities are interconnected and we need to do this together, when people are exhausted, their response is: "Yeah, I understand. But how can I possibly make a difference?"

Then, you pile on top of that all these pre-existing problems and all the things lacking in public education. Counselors, for example: The recommended student-to-counselor ratio is 250-1. As I mentioned before, in Arizona, it's 903-1. This was already a problem before the pandemic. We have the highest class sizes in the nation here in Arizona. When I was still teaching, I had thirty-four kids in my science classroom! I had never experienced that before. My classes in Chicago never even got close to that number. How do you socially distance in a class of thirty-four kids? You don't! *And*, on top of the counselor shortage, there's also no teachers. We have the biggest shortage of teachers and substitutes. Even if you wanted to try to divide up the classes and provide smaller class sizes, there are simply not enough teachers to make that happen. What's happening now is they're just taking any warm body. In some districts, you can basically sign up to be a substitute as long as you get a fingerprint card and have a GED . . . or an associate's, or a bachelor's. You don't even have to have any certifications or education training, because they're gonna continue forcing educators back into the classroom, and they need as many bodies as they can get.

They don't care . . . they don't care. All these public officials are gonna say, "We have to think about 'learning loss' and 'the achievement gap!'"

These are lies. "Learning loss" is a lie. We're in a pandemic! How are you measuring that "learning loss" right now? What I wish people understood is: There's nothing objective or permanent about these things. The standards we teach to, the goals we set for students—these are social constructs that we have decided to apply to certain grades and age groups, which means we can change them. We can modify the things kids need and learn. That's what we do best as educators.

There's also the lack of nurses. Could you imagine if we had a nurse in every school? Could you imagine the effort we could accomplish here to get people vaccinated in our communities if we had a nurse in every school who was trained to deliver the vaccine? Well, we don't have nurses at every school, and that was pre-COVID. And, of course, there's the health care system in general. Imagine if we had Medicare for All right now! But the U.S. won't even guarantee health care to people *in a pandemic*. Maybe they're asymptomatic, maybe they're symptomatic, but parents and students are forced to come to school when they shouldn't because they don't have the money to go to the doctor. Now we're all risking our lives because of a basic lack of health care in this country.

And what about food insecurity and unemployment? What about eviction notices, now that the eviction moratorium has expired? We've got all these serious systemic problems converging, and you're gonna talk about reopening schools for students' mental health? How are you going to care about their mental health now when you don't care if they have food or a place to live? If we cared about students' mental health, then we should be tackling evictions and helping people. I can't tell you how many GoFundMe campaigns I see now for students who are going to lose their housing.

So, yes, all of these pre-existing problems that existed in the public education system have been exacerbated by COVID. We all knew that would happen, but no one listens to teachers. Not one decision-maker listens to us. Even our unions don't listen to us. Our union says they're membership driven. Then why did we have to create these external structures ourselves in order to push you in the right direction? All of this has been laid bare for the nation to see. The economy depends on our labor. But you know what? *We* own our labor, not them—not our principals, not our districts. We own it, and we decide what we want to do with our labor and whether or not to withhold our labor. That's the message we're trying to get through here. I have no strong thoughts or feelings about any of this, as you can tell.

Max: [Laughs.] Yeah, clearly! I've got to pull it out of ya, I guess. Why don't you tell readers how you really feel, Rebecca?

Rebecca: [Laughs.]

Max: I could genuinely talk to you about this all day, but I don't want to take liberties with your time. By way of rounding us out, I wanted to end on that question of unity you were talking about. Right now, politically, this is obviously an important question. But it's also something that I want people to think about when they pick this book up in the future, when they read it and try to put themselves in the shoes of those of us who are living through this now . . . or when they try to remember who they were when they were experiencing this pandemic themselves.

Like you said before, it's been really depressing, and depressingly predictable, to see all the different ways that people in power and powerful institutions—the media, state houses, Washington D.C., the bosses, mayors, the school boards, etc.—have constantly goaded and encouraged us, as a population, to partake in this divide-and-conquer free-for-all. But there have been pointed moments of unity, too, right? I think a lot of us may forget that, in the beginning of this pandemic, there were moments when people were banging pots and pans on their balconies and out of their windows to celebrate frontline health care workers . . .

Rebecca: Right!

Max: There was also a lot of public support for getting workers the PPE they need and securing the hazard pay they deserve. There was even growing support for providing emergency health care for everyone . . . because, shit, if you don't see the need for universal health care during a deadly pandemic, I don't think you ever will. And yet, the longer this pandemic has gone on, the more the months have piled up, the easier it's been for our hopes to shrivel up—and for that potential for collective unity to kind of dissolve into the individual struggle for survival. It's like our immediate and localized needs eventually take over our collective needs. Or that's how it feels, at least. But, like you said, those are the outcomes this system is designed to produce. We live in a society that doesn't guarantee or supply basic human necessities like housing, health care, childcare, etc. And so, *because* we live in such an unjust society where these necessities are not secured for everyone, we—as human beings, as workers—are forced to prioritize securing those things for ourselves over securing them for working people everywhere. We are forced to worry about keeping a roof over our own heads instead of collectively coming together to hold the people in power and the institutions that have failed us accountable for their actions. And they *have* failed us . . . they have failed us immeasurably.

If you could speak to people in the future, what can we tell them this pandemic has taught us about the importance of unity—unity among educators, and between educators and the broader community? In years to come, when someone picks this book up, what takeaway lessons would you want them to learn from your experience as an organizer among educators?

Rebecca: When I think of all the random conversations I have—whether they take place in social media spaces, organizing spaces, parent spaces, interview spaces, etc.—the one thing that I always come back to is the lack of unity we have *as* workers. We *are* the working class. And understanding that, having that consciousness, means recognizing that there is a capitalist class: They're the one-percenters. They have more wealth and power than the rest of us. They have built these systems that oppress and divide us, and that is very much intentional.

As an education worker, I keep thinking about how striving for and building unity in the education space—even just here, in Arizona—is such a massive undertaking. What I mean by that is: Whether you're a bus driver, a paraprofessional, a classified worker, a cafeteria worker, etc.—if you work in the education system, you're with us. That's our unity. That's why we're called "Educators United" instead of "Teachers United." That was a very conscious choice on our part, so we could build that unity and have wall-to-wall organizing in education. But we just don't have that kind of unity between segments of the working class in this country. That's why it's so sad and frustrating when I hear, even among educators, people pushing back against raising the federal minimum wage to $15 an hour. This has been such a long fight, and *finally* it looks like demands for a $15 minimum wage might possibly be met. But I see educators pitting ourselves against people in our own class and saying, "Well, $15 an hour is what I made as a first-year teacher, and I have a degree!" That sort of mentality, that tendency to compare ourselves and believe we're somehow above or below our fellow workers . . . that needs to change.

To me, the ultimate goal of unity is to unite the working class. Because there *is* a class war going on, it *is* us versus them. But we, the 99 percent, need to understand that we are not at war with each other. That's a really hard shell for people to break out of, especially out here where that mentality is beaten out of people and they think, "I live in a 'right-to-work' state—that means I have no rights." Breaking that barrier was really hard back in 2018. But we did it. And so, whenever I think about unity, I think about how much power we, as a labor movement, will have once we, as workers, realize that we are together in this fight.

The forms that unity can take might look different in different locations, in different struggles, depending on people's different capacities and living conditions, etc., but we are together, nonetheless. And if we're talking about society more broadly, I think one of the most important lessons here is that our communities are interconnected. COVID has made that clearer than ever: This is a transmissible virus that doesn't stay within district or city limits; you can't pretend your communities aren't interconnected. I go to different towns all the time, and this whole idea that we and our schools exist in our own little silos, cut off from the rest of the world, is complete nonsense. I don't know how we can make that shift to thinking of ourselves as one, as a connected community, but we need to. That community unity, that worker unity, is so lacking right now. We need a strong labor movement to counteract that . . . and we're working on it. Like I said, educators, nurses, workers who have continued to push back—we are the vanguard of the labor movement right now. If this pandemic does not convince us that all of us need to unite as workers, what other point in history is going to push us to do that? If not now, then when?

3. Duane "Chili" Yazzie

My name is Duane "Chili" Yazzie and I'm here in Shiprock, Navajo Nation, in New Mexico. I've lived here most of my life, although I was born just west of Flagstaff, Arizona—a little community which was a military depot where my dad was working when I was born. My folks brought me back here to Shiprock when I was about two years old, so I grew up here.

I did some schooling out in Oakland that didn't last long—it was just a little tech school. I had an accident, I came home. Then I went back to Frisco and went through a vocational tech school to learn computer programming and data processing. This was the early 1970s, when computers were just first coming into play. In the spring of 1970, I was inducted into the military, but they didn't pick me because I was hurt at the time from my accident. So, I came home after my schooling in Frisco in spring, 1972. I had done a lot of work before with my dad—he was a house builder. After not being able to find a job in the computer field, I went back to work with him. But the Bureau of Indian Affairs, who had financed my schooling in the Bay Area, felt that all their expense for my training should not go to waste. They took me up to Salt Lake City in the summer of '72 —they took me up and down the valley. I had interviews all over the place, but I never was able to find any kind of work in computers and data processing. It was just such a new field. And I imagine that a brownskin asking for a job in that field wasn't received very well anyway. So, I never got an opportunity to work in that field.

I just came home in the fall of 1972, then I hooked up with a rock-and-roll band out of Albuquerque by the name of XIT . . . you can Google XIT and find some of our stuff there. I was in the band for two years, and I ended up coming back home in late 1974 and continued working with my dad. The summer of '74 is when we had some major marches and protests against the city of Farmington, which is just thirty miles from us. I've been regarded as an activist for Indigenous causes and Indigenous rights since 1969, so I was very much involved with the marches in '74—at times we generated over one thousand and up to two thousand people. It was a boycott and a protest march against mistreatment of our people. That summer, some of the White kids there at the high school had murdered three Navajo men—that's what sparked our protests. We marched for seven consecutive Saturdays, just basically shutting the place down. That was the highpoint of my 1974 era.

Going into 1975, I continued to participate in different protest activities. Then, in July of 1975, the local community government reached out to me. We call our local governments "chapters," which are, of course, subunits of our big Navajo tribal government. Each chapter has a set of elected officials, and I was asked to run for what we call the chapter secretary. And I won. I did my four years there, then I continued working with the chapter for two more years. In '82 I came on staff with then-chairman Peterson Zah in Window Rock, the chairman of the Navajo Nation. I was there for four years, serving on the executive staff. Toward the end of that term, I ran for Navajo Nation Council (our legislative body), and I won. I went into the Council in 1986 and served for two terms; that was a good time. In my second term I ended up becoming the chairman of the Budget Finance Committee, which is regarded as the most powerful committee, and that was good. After that term, I came home and just basically did some consulting work for four years.

In 2000, I ran for the chapter presidency here in my community, and I won. I served two terms, up through 2008, and then I went back into doing consulting work with different chapters. Then, in 2012, I came back into the presidency, and I just finished out my term here this past month, in January. All in all, I served my community, my Navajo Nation, for about forty-five years. That turned into my life—my career, so to speak.

Now I'm just here at home, in Shiprock. I like to tout my credentials: I say, "I'm a grandpa, I'm a farmer, I'm an Earth defender, and a community leader."

I'm home now, just doing what we need to do around the place with our farm. Near the end of 2019, we started bringing a group of farmers together with the idea of participating in what we call the Farm-to-School Program with our school districts here, providing fresh produce to the kids and so on. So, we started organizing that; then, as we went into March 2020 or so, this crazy pandemic hit, and that really diverted our focus. The produce that we were generating was needed by the relief agencies, so we started supplying produce to the area relief agencies and to most of the pueblos along the Rio Grande Valley here in New Mexico. And so, we were very busy all summer and into the fall, to the end of the harvest season, with that activity. We did good. And the primary focus of our group, which we call the Shiprock Traditional Farmers' Cooperative, is to revitalize farmlands that sit idle here in the Shiprock community. We have approximately 5,800 acres and, sadly, in recent years we've farmed maybe one thousand acres—the rest of the lands lay fallow. So we're intent on revitalizing much of those acres in order to become a major player in fresh produce for our region, for our people, and for the regional market.

We have great plans to become a mass producer—we want to get into canning produce and food preservation. You know, some of the advantages that we have come from the fact that we've been farmers for centuries. We have food-preservation processes that we carry on, techniques that were developed before there were refrigerators. And then, we also have the value-added products: We have so many different products we can make out of our corn, for instance. We're already a major producer with those value-added products. And, for sure, we want to do, and we are absolutely doing, organic production. We're also very strong on regenerative farming and the whole effort to protect the Earth, to make the best use of the Earth and all of her elements that we have been blessed with. That's where we're at right now. We have a great group of traditional farmers here, and all this activity is keeping me very busy.

At our board meetings . . . well, let me explain that. We call the "board" the Council of Naat'áanii . . . "Naat'áanii" is our Navajo word for "leader." So, we have our council meetings and we conduct them in our own language. As far as the council membership goes, there's seven people . . . and five of them are women. We recognize the great significance and importance of having women in leadership, especially in this realm, where we're working the land and perpetuating our intrinsic relationship with the Earth, which is obviously regarded as a female deity. We call her Earth Mother. And the water, too—water also has a female designation. This all goes way, way back into the eons, back to our original teachings, our original instructions as a people, which tell us that, at the time of creation—and I certainly believe this—there were four instances of creation, not just one.

At the time of the creation of the four colors of man, each was given a principal responsibility in life: The Black People were given guardianship over the essence of water, which, again, is female. The Yellow People were given understanding of the air, and the air is of a male designation. The White People were given guardianship over fire. And we, the Red People, were given the role and responsibility of nurturing and caring for the Earth. Those are the four elements of our life. And we, as Indigenous peoples, from the Arctic Circle down to the tip of South America—we certainly carry on our ceremony, our songs, our stories, in order to perpetuate our responsibility in life, to maintain that balance the best we can, even in this topsy turvy, crazy world we live in now.

And to be fair, we do know that there are Black tribes in Africa who also maintain that ceremony for the water. We know that over in Tibet there are Tibetan monks carrying on their ceremony 24/7, and the focus of their ceremony is the air. We also understand that somewhere over there in Switzerland, or thereabouts, there are White people who maintain that sacred guardianship of fire. Certainly, those ceremonies are very deliberate, and we're all intended to do this work in concert to maintain the equilibrium and the balance of the Earth. But somewhere along the way, people got greedy, and selfish, and jealous. Unfortunately, White folks tell their own story about the apple, the serpent, and Eve in the garden, which is where the negative, the great sin, the evil began. And of course, as we know, it's these teachings of Western thought and technology that predominate, that pervade society, the economy, and so-called social progress—and we're certainly feeling the negative repercussions of that. And so, as the Red Tribe, all we can do is continue to do our part in maintaining that balance the best way we can, and that all works in sync with our effort to do our farming, to improve our agriculture, and to feed the people. So, Max, that is pretty much a brief overview of who Chili Yazzie is.

Max: Man, this is such a rich and incredible history, and I thank you so much for sharing it with me. There was something you said earlier on when you were laying out your own history that really caught my ear, and I wanted to ask you more about it. You mentioned that, back in the '70s, you were really into computers—and that was at a time when computers, like, took up an entire room, right? [Laughs.] Was there something about computers that really spoke to you or drew your interest? Were you a nerdy computer kid growing up?

Chili: No, I was just a very average, rowdy kid—probably below-par academically. I couldn't say why I was drawn to computers. I suppose it just piqued my interest and I wanted to understand the process and technology of it. In some ways, even though I've never had a job in that field, I think studying computers really gave me insight into the workings of the Western mind. I imagine it was intended for me to get that exposure at that age, so . . .

Max: Isn't that sort of connected to a crucial struggle that happened there in Shiprock? Wasn't the Fairchild incident related to computers somehow?

Chili: That happened in February of 1975.[3] The Fairchild semiconductor plant was set up here. At one point, they were employing over one thousand people, working 24/7, manufacturing microchips, etc. My mom—she was one of the workers there. But what happened there was Fairchild, just like any other mega-corporation, wanted to milk as much profit as they could from the plant. They had very low wages; they really took advantage of the people here. The plant was in the Navajo Nation and Fairchild abused this federal program where the feds would put up, like, half the money for salaries and benefits for the first six months people were employed. They would bring people in through that program, basically pay them half wages, and then, after six months, they'd push them out the door and bring in a new group. That was a misuse of the people. And, as has always been the case with the hierarchy of corporations like Fairchild, they reserved the boardroom for themselves—the

3 In late February of 1975, twenty armed members of the American Indian Movement (AIM) seized control of a semiconductor assembly plant on the Navajo reservation in Shiprock, New Mexico. The plant, which operated twenty-four hours a day, was leased to the Fairchild Camera and Instrument Corporation but owned by the Navajo Tribal Council. Led by AIM treasurer Larry Anderson, the group occupied the plant to protest Fairchild's exploitative labor practices, poor health care, and to demand the immediate rehiring of 140 Navajo workers who had recently been laid off.

locals and people of color weren't very welcome. That was the case here: They wouldn't work with us to come up with a solution, and people here started expressing concerns about that.

Pretty soon there were really loud discussions happening, and that all culminated with the armed takeover of the plant by a group that had formed during the marches in '74—that group was called the Coalition for Navajo Liberation. That group and the American Indian Movement—they came in to take over the plant. I was not involved. I knew the thing was happening but I excused myself, so I didn't participate in that takeover. The end result was that Fairchild said, "To heck with y'all. We're leaving town." And they left. That was a bad experience for our community.

Max: That whole story just . . . it just crystallizes so clearly how this system works, right? From Fairchild using these loopholes to exploit Navajo workers and pay them less, to the company just closing the plant and uprooting without any sort of community representation in their decision making or any accountability to the people there. It's just such a gross and sadly familiar tale . . .

Chili: Yeah, absolutely.

Max: And I guess it also shows how the forms of organization that you've already mentioned—from the council government to the work you're doing with the Shiprock Traditional Farmers' Cooperative—are very much not structured the way companies like Fairchild are, and for good reason! Maybe giving private, hierarchical, unaccountable corporations so much power over our lives and our world is *not* such a good idea . . . but what do I know? Anyway, I want to ask you more about the council, the cooperative, and the response to COVID-19. But before we do that, I couldn't let this pass, because it's such an interesting detail: *You used to tour with a rock band?* What was that like? And when did you, Chili, get a little less rambunctious and settle down? How did you go from touring with a rock band to getting involved in council government?

Chili: Well, the American Indian Movement began in Wisconsin, or somewhere out there, in 1968. The AIM phenomenon came to Shiprock in the summer of 1969, and I was on board with it. Getting involved with the American Indian Movement at the time certainly exposed me to a lot of issues that Native peoples were contending with. That's been my ideological makeup ever since.

When I came back from Salt Lake in the summer of '72, I came across this group called XIT. It was the first time I heard their album, which was called *Plight of the Redman*. As the name suggests, the album was a chronology of our time as Native people since Columbus. It was a great exposé of the plight of Indigenous peoples here in the hemisphere. So it just fit, you know? It fit who I was and what my beliefs were at the time, so I had to join. And all of our music was concept music—we were regarded as the soundtrack of the movement. At the time, there was a great surge of Indian activism; all across the spectrum, people were resisting, rebelling, revolting, protesting. When I was in Frisco, I was there when Alcatraz[4] first started happening, then there were the Black Panthers over in Oakland, and in downtown Frisco and Berkeley you had all these massive marches against the war. I saw all that. So, for me to become a member of XIT—it was a natural fit. It wasn't a divergence from my life, my outlook. It was just another very comfortable activity that was in alignment with who I was and what I wanted to do and say. It was a great opportunity, and I never regret it. We had our wild times, as rock-and-roll people do, but our music—there was a message to it. In fact, it was called "the Gospel of the Redman." We were regarded as radicals, a protest group, so we never got the kind of play in downtown America that Redbone did. You know Redbone, with their hit "Come and Get Your Love?"

Max: Yeah.

Chili: . . . Redbone was our nemesis.

Max: [Laughs.]

---

4 On November 20, 1969, under the group name Indians of All Tribes (IOAT), eighty-nine Indigenous men, women, and children occupied Alcatraz Island in San Francisco, California. Reaching a peak of 400 occupants at one point, Indigenous peoples and families held the island for nineteen months to protest colonial genocide and repression of Native Americans and to demand the return of Tribal lands.

Chili: They did commercial stuff, with some Native themes of course. We actually played back-to-back with Redbone on several occasions. If it was for a Native audience, you know, we could talk to the Native people—we could communicate with them. We always ended up getting a better review than Redbone did when we played with them. But yeah, all in all, playing with XIT was a good fit. There was no interruption of my general quest in life. So, it was . . . it all worked out well.

Max: It's awesome that you got to have that experience. Like you said, you're young, there's a lot going on, you've got a lot to say—why not seize the opportunity? And, you know, when I talk to folks who had these types of experiences in their youth, usually they'll say that it was family that sort of brought them down to earth a bit. When you came home from being a rock-and-roller, did you come back to settle down and start a family, or did that happen later?

Chili: The group kind of drifted apart around December of 1974. I came home around that time, in early '75, and was working here and there. Apart from the marches, things got kind of quiet. So, yeah, Betsy and I got married in April 1975—we've been together forty-six years now.

Max: Congratulations! I remember you saying earlier . . . let me see, I wrote it down . . . that you're proud to call yourself a grandfather, a farmer, an Earth protector, and a community leader. Those are all really beautiful things to be. Tell me a bit about your family. How many grandchildren do you and Betsy have?

Chili: We've got three kids and nine grandchildren—and two great grandchildren.

Max: Wow! That's amazing, man. And I hear that you have quite a story about the day one of your children was born, is that right?

Chili: Yeah. In 1975—late '75—we had our first child. And one day in 1978, June 27, while I was the chapter secretary there at the chapter house, Betsy was two weeks past due with our son Lance. That afternoon

I was driving to Farmington, the town thirty miles away, to get my license renewed or something like that. Now, in my earlier years I did a lot of hitchhiking, to Albuquerque, to Salt Lake City, all over the area. So I know what hitchhiking is about, and I would always pick up hitchhikers—didn't ask questions. That afternoon I was leaving town, heading to Farmington, and there was a hitchhiker sitting there against the signpost. He was a tall White boy. You've seen Clint Eastwood's spaghetti westerns like *The Good, the Bad, and the Ugly*, where he has his poncho and his floppy hat?

Max: Yeah.

Chili: This guy was duded up like that. Anyway, I stopped for him, and he got in with his big backpack, and we proceeded to drive up to Farmington. I was just in my own world, playing my Creedence Clearwater music. He generated what little conversation we had about where he was coming from, where he was going, and so on. He offered me some whiskey, which I declined two times. And there, outside of Farmington, about five miles west of Farmington, he said he needed to go to the bathroom, so he asked me to pull over so he could take a piss. So I did, right there on top of the hill coming into Farmington. I pull off the road, maybe thirty yards or so back from the highway, and put the car in park.

I was waiting for the guy to get out, but he didn't move. I looked over at him, and he's just sitting there staring at me. And of course he has his poncho on, so I don't know what's under there. All of a sudden, the greatest impact that a person can feel just hit me. I've been fist-punched really hard a few times, I played football and all that, but this was unlike anything I'd ever felt. The whole world changed right there. My perception . . . everything turned brown, like a bad sandstorm. Turns out, under his poncho, he was aiming his pistola at me—for no reason. I was just giving the guy a lift, we didn't have any words or anything like that. The police said that small-time crooks like him have a coming-out moment—they go "big time" at some point. And on that day he was going big time. I just happened to be in the way.

So he shot me, and it just crashed me into the door. I look back at him and, you know, it's just like in the movies: There's smoke coming out of that little hole in his poncho. I cussed at him, threw a few expletives at him, and he shot me again. I knew this guy wasn't gonna give me no kind of slack, so I suppose my survival instinct kicked in and I opened the door. I knew my arm was hurt really bad, so I just grabbed it, held it to myself, got out of the car, and ran. I ran about twenty to twenty-five feet, and the whole time I'm thinking, "Just don't shoot me in the back." Finally I stopped, turned around, and I saw him peel out in my ride. It was a hot day, June 27 . . . I looked at myself and I was just streaming, streaming blood. My instinct was telling me to get to the hospital. So I walked to the highway and there I am, a bloody mess, and I'm hitchhiking to the hospital with my left thumb. Three cars with White folks passed by—guess they didn't want me to get their cars messy. Finally, this old pickup truck came chugging up the hill and the guy recognized me. He pulled back around, pulled me into the truck, and got me to the hospital.

They started prepping me for surgery and I told them to call Betsy, so she came up to the E.R. and, of course, she was very large. I was in surgery all night—probably from like six o'clock to four or five in the morning. They worked me over all night. The first bullet hit my arm bone straight on. It shattered the bullet, shattered the bone, and it all blew inside me. They had to take part of my lung off because it was pretty damaged. The second bullet came into my lower side, and it went all the way through my middle part. Turns out he shot me with a .44 Magnum . . .

Max: Jesus.

Chili: I brag around now. I say, "I survived a .44 Magnum two times, point blank."

Max: [Laughs.] Man, I would too! That'll get you a free drink anywhere you go.

Chili: Yup. So, they finally got done with me in surgery. Next morning, I'm waking up, they have me on morphine and all kinds of junk, but I'm conscious. I can tell what's happening—and the doctor brought in this little bundle. It was my baby boy, still wet from birth. While I was getting worked over in surgery Betsy had gone into labor down the hall, and she delivered our boy. The doctor said, "You know, we don't expect you to live. You have less than a fifty-fifty chance. At least you should see your boy." That's all I needed, apparently. I was in the hospital for thirty days, then I got out. Lance, our son—he rescued me from the brink.

Max: Damn, that's incredible, man. God, what an experience. I don't even know what to say. That is wild, though—you and Betsy in the same hospital, right down the hall from each other . . .

Chili: [Laughs.]

Max: Well, speaking of hospitals and health crises, I was wondering if we could turn our focus to this crazy reality of COVID-19 that we've all been experiencing over the past year. I'm sure readers will have seen the news coming out of Navajo Nation, which got hit really hard by the pandemic in 2020, but there are also stories coming out as we speak about how the Navajo Nation has had one of the most successful systems for administering vaccines. Could you talk a bit about how you, your family, and your community have experienced this pandemic?

Chili: I guess people like us—we try to rationalize things, to find the root causes. We've done that here, and I've done that myself. The conclusion that I've made is that, because of the great abuse of the Earth, she's basically rebelling against the mistreatment. I write, you know—I write a lot of stuff. And in one of my writings, I talked about the fact that COVID-19 is a thing of nature. It's not anything mechanical—it's alive. What I say is: It's alive with death. To me, it's a great discipline whip of the Earth, basically punishing the people of the world for the mistreatment, for letting things go to this extreme. And it doesn't discriminate, you know? It's a very democratic kind of situation we have with this virus. Nobody's exempt.

Having said that (I wanted to give you my perspective first so it would give some context for everything else), we got hit with this thing back in March or so, and we basically went undercover. I've been mostly home all year—only going out when I have to. I'm glad to have gotten my shots here just the other day. But I guess some people—they refuse to recognize the seriousness of situations like that. That's how it was here at the outset of our response to COVID, at least with our tribal leadership. We did start with these lockdowns quite early, and we still have them. We're locked down every weekend, for fifty-seven hours, and we have a nightly curfew. The response from our nation has been pretty strong. But the spread was already happening here and the infection rate, unfortunately, was pretty high. And it spread for different reasons. Being lax with recognizing the seriousness of the situation—that was one reason. But the thing is: Our life conditions really amplified the seriousness and the need. Some of that stems from the mistreatment we've gotten as a people of color, because we are so economically disadvantaged. We were thrust into this new world, new society, new economics, and we've been at a disadvantage for many, many generations. And, unfortunately, many people aren't able to deal with that. So, yeah, we have high rates of alcoholism and drug abuse—people trying to contend with these circumstances. Then, because of our lack of economics and so on, there's a critical housing shortage here. In a lot of cases, you'll find three generations living in one house, and oftentimes those houses are dilapidated to begin with. That remains one of the concerns for our health people and our government people: How do we isolate people, how do we put individuals in quarantine, when there's no place to isolate them?

So, it hit us really hard. My family—we had skirmishes with it. Two of my daughters have no option but to work with the public; their work situations are such that they've both had people around them who were infected, and they've had to be quarantined for a time. But, in general, we're all good. All my kids, all my grandkids—we're doing good. Although it has hit really close. Just this past Saturday, for instance, we buried my son-in-law's father. We've lost some very close people: extended family members, people I work with . . . we lost one of our tribal presidents just last week.

Max: My God. I'm so sorry.

Chili: Yeah . . . When this thing started happening, those of us in leadership . . . we understand that the need is great. We know that many homes and families lack the resources and the ability to respond to the situation. That's why, here in Shiprock, I helped found the Northern Diné COVID Relief Effort. "Diné" is the name that we have for ourselves, rather than "Navajo." I worked with that group for three or four months until I moved on to this farming venture that we've got going now. But yeah, I know that even Dr. [Anthony] Fauci recognized the success, if you can call it that, of the Navajo Nation in bringing the continued spread of the disease under control, at least within reasonable measure.

But, you know, I do think that this situation really portends great catastrophe. We have food being trucked in every week, which is distributed to families. And when all this food comes in, one thing I wonder about is: Is there a limitless supply? Will we start experiencing shortages here at some point? Because of all these circumstances, because of our economic and social conditions, we're at a great disadvantage as a people. If those shortages happen, what do we do? What will our people do? It's with that big thought in mind that we're doing what we're doing with our agriculture. We can't depend on the supermarket permanently; we're going to have to feed ourselves. That's what we're doing now with the Shiprock Traditional Farmers' Cooperative. We're brand new, so we're certainly still in the building process. We've been fortunate to get some funding—small grants here and there—but to get to the level that we want to get to, to test our limits and our capability and our potential, we will absolutely need greater resources to make that happen. We're in a building process and in much need of support. Any help people can offer us is really appreciated.

4. Willy Solis

My name is Willy Solis. I'm forty-two years old, and I live in Denton, Texas, which is a suburb of Dallas.

Max: Are you originally from Texas?

Willy: Yeah, born and raised in Dallas-Fort Worth. It's a pretty large city—a nice, comfortable place for us to grow up. Since we grew up here, my family wanted to stay here. I decided to raise my kids here too.

Max: What was the path that led you to getting involved in gig work? I ask because I think about this kind of thing a lot, especially as it pertains to my own family. My dad drove for Uber, my mom drove for Uber, my brother drove for Lyft for a while, and he's also done a lot of delivery driving. I often find myself trying to remember the timeline of events that led to the so-called "gig economy," and then I try to map our experience onto that timeline. I remember when companies like Uber were just popping up and the whole gig model was still a very new thing—I think that was mainly in the early 2010s, in the wake of the recession. How did you experience the emergence of the gig economy? Where were you when you first started to notice these companies and services cropping up? And when did you yourself eventually get involved in that kind of work?

Willy: My history—my upbringing and my career path—has been a little all over the place, to be honest. But a big part of the work I was doing before involved a lot of travel. It was when I was doing all that traveling that I first started coming into contact with these gig companies and the gig economy in general. I used Uber first as a consumer. There were a lot of instances when I needed to get from point A to point B, and that was right around the time Uber and Lyft were starting to become really popular. I had already started to hear from friends and family that they were doing rideshare driving and getting involved in gig work. This was back in 2009–2010. But I really started paying attention around 2011 and 2012; I was traveling quite a bit then. By that point, Uber seemed to be popping up everywhere, so that's when I really took notice.

Max: And what was the transition like for you? When did you go from seeing this as a service you could use as a consumer to thinking about it as a viable source of income? I know a lot of folks out there now rely on gig work as their primary source of income, but many probably first got involved in gig work thinking it could be a supplement to their other jobs. That's how it was sold to us, right? It was always pitched as a kind of "side hustle" to earn some extra cash—that's where the "gig" name comes from. What was the process like for you? How did you go from seeing this as a viable source of secondary income to potentially even a primary job? And could you also talk a bit about what gig work offered you that was attractive? What sold you on it?

Willy: Like I said before, because of all the traveling I was doing, I was getting a lot of exposure to the gig economy, and I would see these people all over the place making a little bit of extra income. Every time I got into another Uber car I would ask the driver questions: "How much do you actually make with this job? Is it a good source of income?" All that kind of stuff. So, I had generally started poking and prodding, talking to actual Uber and Lyft drivers and other gig workers, for a while. I really didn't think about becoming a gig worker myself, though, until it was borne out of necessity in 2019.

At the time, I was in a transition period with my career: I was closing down my business. I had been an independent contractor since 2008, so I understand what it means to be independent. Running my own residential construction business taught me what true profit/loss is and how expenses impact profitability. I also learned the management of risk and asset allocation. After just a few short weeks of doing gig work it became clear I was not truly independent.

Uber, Lyft, and gig companies in general—they seemed to be offering low barriers to entry, which meant that I could quickly jump into doing the work and bring in some income. I decided to test it out, to see if I could use it as a bridge to the next adventure in my career. I started looking through and studying the different gig apps that were available at the time, and I started applying to quite a few of them, including Instacart and Shipt. I signed up for Uber Eats too. I preferred making deliveries to driving people from point A to point B. I'm more of a loner, so I didn't really want anybody in my car.

For me, the main things I was looking for with gig work were: that it would give me the flexibility I needed; that there was a low entry point, so I could jump in and out whenever I needed to; and, basically, that I could make it revolve around what I needed. My understanding, and the way it was sold to me, was that this is your own little, independent business. You'll be able to make your own hours, your own decisions, etc. Having run a large business since 2008, I figured this would be a great opportunity for me. But, yeah, from the beginning the intent behind getting into gig work was always to make it a bridge to whatever came next. It was supposed to be temporary. I was only supposed to do it for a month or two.

At the time, I was actually trying to get my license in Florida for construction work, which is a very long and time-consuming process. By that point, though, I was on the back end of the licensing process, so I anticipated being finished with my Florida work soon enough, but that kind of fell through. That's when I realized I was going to need a new full source of income. "I need to figure this gig economy stuff out," I thought, "because now I'm basically going to have to utilize this work to make a living, to be my bread and butter." I kind of ended up getting stuck in the gig economy prior to the pandemic, and I've had to figure this thing out as I go along. One of the hardest things to do was understand that this whole gig economy, which was sold as a flexible, independent business, is actually far from it. The more I recognized that, the more I could see how people got caught in this cycle where they remained stuck in the gig economy and couldn't get out. People often say, "Oh, why don't you just quit and go find another job?" Sometimes it's just not that easy, especially when you have very limited opportunities. You'll be looking for different avenues to advance your career, become self-sufficient, and make a substantial living, but sometimes there aren't any.

I ended up realizing very quickly that I could make some pretty good money with Shipt.[5] The other gig apps were starting to let me down—the ways they were structured made it really difficult to bring in decent money. So I started sticking with Shipt, and I learned as much as I could about it. That's what drew me into a situation where I eventually found myself becoming an organizer with Shipt workers.

Max: Man, even just hearing you talk now about why this work was attractive, it really resonates. Like you said, being more of a loner and preferring to be on your own, doing deliveries and such is kind of the perfect gig for you, right? That's got me thinking of my days as a pizza delivery guy, back when I was delivering for a pizzeria called Zito's in Anaheim. The things you're describing—that was my favorite part of the job. I could hop in my car and be on my own, and it was great. This was back in the day when we still had to print out the Google Maps route from the office computer instead of having smartphones navigating for us. I would pick up a delivery ticket, grab the map printout, put all the food in those insulated red bags, and head out. And this was Southern California, so I'd be driving on the freeways, I'd have my window down, the music would be blaring, I'd smoke some cigarettes [laughs]. That shit ruled. There was just something so attractive about doing the work that I needed to do but having the freedom to do it on my own, in my own car. That's why it's so easy to imagine that, if you have these gig companies trying to capitalize on the allure of that kind of work environment, that's going to be very attractive to a lot of people. It makes a lot of sense that people would see this not only as a viable source of income but a job that they would actually *like* to do.

But then, something kind of sets in—I could hear this in the story that you were telling, and it's something I've heard from so many friends and other folks who have done gig work. You just start to get this creeping sense that you're not as alone as you thought you were . . . that you don't have as much freedom as you were told you have. You start to see how

5 Shipt is an app- and web-based delivery service owned by Target Corporation. Relying on "gig workers" who receive, shop, and deliver customer orders, Shipt offers same-day delivery from various retailers in the U.S.

much power that app on your phone has to dictate where you go and what you do on the job.

Willy: Right. And that's really where the problem is. Having done so much work previously as an independent contractor, I fully understood then that every single day, every single thing I did, every action I took—everything rested on my own shoulders. If something didn't get done, or if it was done incorrectly, it was my fault, and I had to figure out how to fix it. With gig work, it's totally different. You are not independent in any way, shape, or form. You *believe* that you are, at first, but as soon as something unexpected happens you have to rely entirely on what the app tells you to do. Or, if you call in to Shopper Support—or Driver Support, or whatever the app's hotline for gig workers is—then they dictate every action that you do. The service that you want to provide to the consumer is really mitigated or controlled by what these gig companies want. And, I mean, I recognize that their names and their brands are on the line too. Having run a business, I can relate. You want to make sure that your brand isn't tarnished by a bad experience that a customer had with a driver or somebody else not providing the best quality of service. I understand that aspect of it. The problem, though, is that when these companies start exercising that level of control, when they're dictating just about everything you do and how you respond to every situation, that's where you lose any semblance of independence. And a lot of the things you do as a gig worker do require independent thinking—they require you to be able to make decisions on the spot in order to solve a problem or address a situation. That should really be the responsibility of the driver, or the shopper, or whatever their title is: It should fall on our shoulders. We should be able to decide if we're going to go the extra mile, or if we're just going to provide the basic service that we're contracted for. There are situations, for instance, when I need to take a different route than the one the app is telling me to take, or go to a different store that's a little bit closer. For these companies to tell me that I have to drive across town when I can clearly see on the map that the customer's house is located much closer to me and that there's a closer store nearby—same brand, same everything—it just doesn't make sense. However, if I don't go across town like the app is telling me to, then at that point I can get myself into trouble and get deactivated. So, the independence that you feel you have with gig work quickly goes away once you start doing this on a daily basis.

Max: Let's talk a little bit about that day-to-day reality and what it's like on the job for you and other shoppers for services like Shipt and Instacart. Could you talk about what a "normal day" or a "normal week" on the job entailed before the pandemic? I know that, even before COVID-19 hit, there were a lot of issues that you and your fellow Shipt shoppers experienced and were trying to address with Shipt's parent company [Target Corporation]. What did work look like for you before the pandemic? And what sorts of issues were arising that made you feel you had to speak up?

Willy: Before the pandemic started there were quite a few issues. The primary one had to do with the fact that whenever there was a problem with a card not working—we use a prepaid credit card provided by Shipt—or if an order wasn't processing in the app, or if you had any difficulty getting ahold of the customer, or if the address was incorrect, you'd have to reach out to Shopper Support and try to get some assistance. Now, the problem was that, when you tried to call Shopper Support, you would be on hold for anywhere between twenty minutes to a couple of hours. In some situations, when you got closer to Thanksgiving and Christmas, you were looking at more than a couple of hours. Sometimes it would take a day or two to get a response. Try to imagine going to the store and shopping a full order: You have a full basket or cart of groceries, you've got perishable goods that have to be refrigerated, or they have to be accounted for in some other way in regards to food safety. You're trying to get the app to work, or you're trying to get the card to process so you can pay at the register. You're standing there with people behind you, looking over your shoulder, wondering when you're going to get out of their way. That's a very lonely feeling. When those situations arise, the only option you have is to pick up the phone and call the Shopper Support line—and when I would call, the situation would just start escalating or kind of snowballing.

We work with these basic parameters, right? Like "on-time delivery"—that's one of the metrics we have on the app that measures our ability to perform services well. These metrics are how they measure us and rate our performance. The other metrics are "customer rating" and "acceptance rate" (i.e., the number of orders you accept when the app sends them to you). These things are really important to us, because they dictate our earning potential. If any of those three ratings is damaged in any way, it affects the kinds of orders that we get and the amount of orders that we get from the Shipt app and it basically puts us lower on the totem pole. So we're very protective of our ratings.

Going back to the store . . . you're standing there, feeling helpless, the card's not working, the app's not working, and you got the store cashier looking at you like, "When are you going to pay?" And you're there on your phone, on hold, and you realize very quickly that nobody's coming to help you—or, if they are, it's going to take a long time. So, you have to excuse yourself at the register, go off to the side, and try to work your way through the troubleshooting process. These situations would happen often, and I'd be standing there, leaning against a wall in the grocery store, and the whole time I'd be wondering, "What is the customer thinking right now? Am I going to be late? Are they going to hurt my rating?" And, sure enough, there were times when I was late with a delivery because the card or app wouldn't work. It would take over twenty to thirty minutes for Shopper Support to get on the phone. Once they finally got on the phone with me, we would work things out pretty quickly. But that whole time you're waiting to get these issues fixed—you're not getting paid for that. On top of that, if an item in the order is temperature sensitive, I have to go to the store employee and say, "Hey, this has been out too long. You guys are gonna have to dispose of it and I'm gonna have to get another one." Obviously, when you're facing that kind of situation, the store managers are not too happy with you.

Because of these issues, I ended up getting dinged on the app a couple of times for being late. It got to the point where I started asking questions on the Facebook groups that Shipt runs. I would say something like, "Hey, this kind of situation happened to me. Can I get any pointers on this kind of thing?" The response was, surprisingly, not very helpful. Instead of pointers, instead of people reaching out and saying, "Hey, maybe you could have done this or that better," I got a lot of put-downs from other Shipt shoppers. Because the community is . . . the only way I can describe it is "very cultish." The tone of everything has to be perfect sunshine and rainbows. If you posted anything negative on these Facebook pages, they would come down on you pretty hard. It was a shopper-policed community I thought I could go to for help, because Shipt said that was where we should go to ask questions, but I quickly found out that that really wasn't where I wanted to ask questions. I didn't appreciate being put down by my fellow shoppers.

Then, the thing I feared would happen did actually happen: I got temporarily deactivated from Shipt in November of 2019. I can honestly sit here today and tell you that the things I got deactivated for were not my fault. There were times when I was running behind and got my ratings dinged, and they were all related to the card not working, or long lines at the grocery store, or some other situation that was beyond my control. I would start my shops really early—I wanted to be ahead of schedule. Remember, this was my only full-time income at that point—I'm trying to protect it as much as I can. When I got deactivated it was very jarring, very shocking, and, to be honest with you, kind of scary. "What am I going to do now?" Yes, this was one app among the others that I was on. At the time I also had Instacart and GrubHub, but the scary part about it is wondering, "If this is happening to me on Shipt, will it happen to me on the other apps?" The answer is: yes. At any time these companies can deactivate you, and you generally have no recourse to try to get back on the app. Luckily for me, Shipt does offer what they call "refresher courses" that you can take if you've been deactivated, which are basically training courses. And when I was taking this training course, I kept thinking in the back of my mind, "Wait a minute, where's the independence? I thought I was supposed to be independent here. Why am I being sent to training to correct my behavior?" Now, I totally agree that we, as shoppers, do need help sometimes, and sometimes we do need some kind of guidance. But to be told that you have to do this in order to be reactivated—that's when I started saying to myself, "This isn't really what independent contractor work is supposed to be like." Companies are not supposed to have that kind of power over you. Nevertheless, I completed the training. I had already reached out to Shipt and told them that these situations weren't my fault, but I only received a canned answer saying that once I completed my training I would be reactivated at some point. It took about a week. For that whole week I was not able to earn income, and that left me in a precarious financial situation. There's not really much you can do in that situation; you've just gotta try and figure out the best way to survive. I did jump on the other apps, but

I quickly realized that these other apps had even *more* control over how much income I could earn than Shipt did. I was really anxious to get back on Shipt, then, because I was able to earn larger payouts overall with larger tips.

Once I finally did get back on Shipt, that's when I started to realize that I really need to protect my ratings, even more than I was before. I became fiercely protective of them. Then in December, when Christmas time came around, you had the same issues with on-time delivery and the same situations with stores being completely packed. This was still pre-COVID, pre-pandemic, so there were a lot of people out shopping in the stores. Getting through that shopper mania was really hard, because not only are you managing the task at hand getting all the items on the customer's list, you also have to manage things that are way outside of your control like excessively long lines—and this is how you're trying to make your living. I tried to learn as much as I could as quickly as I could, but I started to run into the same situations where I would be late for reasons out of my control, and that was very frightening for me. So, I jumped back on the Shipt Facebook groups and I said, "Okay, I'm just going to dive in here and start asking questions. No matter what happens, I'm just going to dig through the responses and try to pick out some wisdom."

Sure enough, once I started asking these questions, I started getting censored. Because they weren't easy questions. I was asking critical questions of the company like, "Why am I not able to reach somebody at Shopper Support within a short period of time instead of sitting on hold?" And, "Why does that delay fall on my shoulders and hurt my rating?" I also asked questions about whether or not I could bring somebody to shop with me as a way of getting around these issues—so, like, they could stand in the long line while I run to get that gallon of milk and come back to the front of the store, then I could check out on time and proceed to my destination. I was quickly told, "No, you cannot co-shop." This got me very curious, because everything that I know about independent contractor work tells me that I can make my own decisions. If I want to bring somebody with me—as long as I know them, they're legal, they've got a background check, and there's no safety concerns—then I should be able to do that.

I decided to read my contract, and the more that I read the contract the more interesting things got. The first thing I realized was that I should have opted out of arbitration within the thirty-day period after your start date. I was like, "Oh, you dummy. You should have done that." But I didn't, and . . . it is what it is. As a result, I am not able to legally challenge any grievances in a court of law or participate in a class-action lawsuit. Instead, I would have to engage in binding arbitration by myself. More importantly, though, I found details in the contract saying that you *can* co-shop—you can actually give a third party access to your app, and you can hire subcontractors to help you. All of this stuff was written out in the contract. But the moment I started asking questions about it in the Facebook groups to someone whom I perceived to be a supervisor . . . they're called "Metro Leads" . . . she quickly told me, "No, you can't co-shop." I would always get referred to this policy manual that Shipt has called the "Shopper Hub." The thing about the Shopper Hub is it has all these policies and rules specifying what you can and can't do, but it's all written very carefully in a language that *implies* very heavily that you *shouldn't* do X or Y, not that you legally *can't* do them. What happens is these policies become like the norm, which is exactly what they want. This is how I like to explain it to people: Through policy, they control us. If we go to court, the contract is written in such a way that it would allow Shipt to say, "No, these people are independent. We don't control them in any way." But when it comes to the policy, that's something totally different. It's the *policy* that specifically says any shopper who's caught co-shopping with somebody else is subject to deactivation. If I'm really an independent contractor, they shouldn't be able to dictate that. Sure, if I want to bring my daughter who's over eighteen years old with me so she can stand in line while I'm going to get the gallon of milk, I'll have to split the money with her and I won't make as much for that shop, but that should be my call. But I can't do that, because the store can report me to Shipt and Shipt will deactivate me for it. That just started seeming more and more unfair to me.

Max: Hearing you describe these things, it's just so clear that, as a gig worker, so much of the responsibility, and so much of the fallout if anything goes wrong, is put entirely on *you*. It's just so . . . punitive. The worker bears all the brunt, right? That's the gig economy in a nutshell. And all of this was going on *before* the pandemic! Let's throw that into the discussion. Through your eyes, as you experienced it, could you talk a bit about how these issues persisted, or how new issues cropped up, as the reality of COVID-19 set in?

Willy: Yeah, a lot of the responsibilities and liabilities do fall on the worker. All the while, the control is really exercised by companies like Shipt. From our perspective, that's where smaller problems start to escalate into bigger problems that wouldn't exist if shoppers were able to exercise our own controls.

Getting closer to the pandemic, one of the things that I started noticing around Christmas time and even going into January was that my tips were actually going down. It wasn't because of the level of service I was providing; in fact, I was actually going well above and beyond what I had done before. And the reason I was going above and beyond was *because* I had noticed that my earnings were going down and I was like, "What is happening?" So, again, I jumped back on those Facebook boards, especially this one Shipt-run group on Facebook called the Shopper Main Lounge, and what I noticed was all these shoppers posting about things they were doing that were really not what we were contracted for. There was one specific post that I remember very well from somebody who was boasting about walking a customer's dog. Other people were boasting about taking out customers' trash, or about buying these gifts they saw at the store and taking them to customers. I started asking questions like, "Why are people doing this? Why would I do that?" I'm already not earning that much, and to lose time taking out somebody's trash or unpacking their groceries in their house or walking their dog, let alone buying some balloons or whatever with my own money—it just didn't make sense to me. It affects how that customer will perceive the next shopper who *doesn't* do those things. For me, being a businessperson, I'm thinking about the bottom line, because I have to. I'm thinking about getting this order in, providing the proper level of service, then moving on to the next one. But going through this process and seeing people posting this kind of stuff, I quickly realized that this was probably why my tips were going down. It's because I'm not doing all this extra stuff. It's not that I'm against being nice to people and trying to go above and beyond—I'm not. I love dogs, I have dogs myself, and I'd love to walk anybody's dog, to be honest with you. It's a lot of fun, it's good exercise, and I really do enjoy it. We have four dogs and I walk them all the time. But to take time out of my work to go do that, to expend that extra energy doing these things—it's just not feasible.

And so, again, I started asking questions on the Facebook groups—and again I was shut down. People were telling me that I was insensitive, and I just got a whole lot of nasty comments that really put me down. I decided to not ask those questions anymore. I didn't like or appreciate the fact that Shipt itself, through their Metro Leads and Facebook group moderators, started deleting my comments just because I asked other shoppers, "Why would you take on the liability of walking somebody's dog? If that dog gets loose, heaven forbid, and gets injured, or if it bites someone, as an independent contractor, you are now liable for whatever happens to that animal." Shipt deleted those comments from their group. And the more that happened, the more alone I felt. While that may not seem like a huge deal, it is. As it is, we are "independent," we are out there by ourselves in the world, we're the ones who have to provide the service, and all that burden falls on our shoulders. So, it really hurts when, the moment we try to reach out to our coworkers to speak about this, they try to shut us down. And so, once we started creeping into February of 2020, that's really when we started ramping up our organizing. I knew these things *do* need to be discussed, but we obviously can't discuss them out in the open. That's why I started reaching out to folks on Facebook Messenger and having private conversations with them. That's really how our organizing was born.

Max: I wanted to ask more about that process of getting your organizing off the ground. Because, like you mentioned, even before these Shipt-run Facebook pages were actively deleting or hiding your comments, there was already a widespread cultural problem that made it difficult to connect with other Shipt shoppers because folks were so judgmental of one another. And, like we were talking about earlier, the gig economy as such really encourages us to believe in this idea that we are *independent* contractors, right? The ideology there really pushes us to feel like we are masters of our own destiny, that the outcomes you get, the money you make, the ratings you get, all depends on you and how hard you're willing to work. I don't want it to sound like I'm saying workers don't have any agency here—we do. But when that ideology roots itself so deeply in your brain, you become totally blind to the ways your agency is being actively *taken* *away* from you, and you punish yourself for things that are entirely out of your control as if they are deeply personal failures. When you're talking to a large group of workers who are in that mindset, it can be very hard to even start that conversation, let alone share your stories openly and vulnerably, for fear that you'll be judged as "lazy" or, you know, "making excuses." These are things I've heard my whole life. I know a ton of friends, family members, and fellow workers who still think this way. How did you get around that? And could you walk through that process of getting around these Facebook pages and connecting with other gig workers directly? What was it like when you were finally able to talk to people on that real, one-to-one level? And how much work did it take on your end to even get to that level and be able to have those conversations in the first place?

Willy: I kind of chuckled at that because it was a tremendous amount of work to get around those Facebook pages. Basically, Shipt had created a culture that I had not seen among workers for any of the other apps. Shipt seemed to be systematically creating these self-policing environments where the shoppers would basically do the dirty work for them—it was the shoppers themselves who would make sure that all the conversations that were happening were nothing but positive. I refer to it as "toxic positivity," because it was just *so* positive no matter what. I'm gonna be straight and honest with you: I'm a very independent thinker, but at the beginning I actually got caught up in it myself. In my mind, I was like, "How do I serve my community more? How do I become a bigger part of this movement that is Shipt?" It just felt like something that I really wanted to be a part of. It was just happy all the time—if you woke up and went out the door, you were happy. If you saw those commercials Shipt was running in February—the ones depicting Shipt shoppers diving into lobster tanks or running across the top of fences—that's how Shipt depicts what we do: always going far above and beyond for the customers.

I remember seeing something in the Shopper Main Hub that said, "If you're out shopping for a customer you know is feeling sick or something like that, you should bring them a balloon." That used to be an explicitly stated policy up until we started talking about it and exposed the fact that Shipt was encouraging this kind of thing, then they removed it. More to the point, though, the culture itself was so . . . the only word I can think of is judgmental. Self-policing was so heavy, nobody really wanted to speak out or question Shipt's policies in any way, shape, or form. So, you started to see these rogue groups that Shipt didn't control popping up on Facebook, and they were an outlet for shoppers to have conversations that were a little outside the realm of what Shipt would allow. At the same time, people were being very careful, because everybody thought and felt that Shipt had infiltrated those groups, which was a legitimate fear. We later found out that it had. We had really high-level people who worked for Shipt (directors of operation, etc.) creeping around in these groups. People were really careful with the words they used and the criticisms they expressed in those groups. In the back of your mind, you always had this fear that if Shipt saw what you say, they would deactivate you. In the end, those rogue groups weren't really a good outlet for people to have substantive discussions.

The more that I noticed that this kind of stuff was happening, and the more that Shipt censored me specifically, the more I began to think, "I don't know if this is what I need to be doing with my life. I may need to go in a different direction, because, financially speaking, this is too much of a vulnerability for me." But that's when I first started hearing rumblings that other people were as unhappy with Shipt as I was—that was in early January. Then January 20 happened. Out of nowhere, Shipt decided to change its pay model in certain cities like Kalamazoo, San Antonio, and Philadelphia. When I heard about the pay change, obviously the first thought in my mind was, "Is this going to happen in Texas? If it is, will it be a good pay change or a bad pay change?" I kind of figured that it wasn't going to be in my favor, but I wanted to make sure that I fully understood it so I could make a plan for myself and my family. The more I dug around, the more I found out that it was not a good change and that it was basically blindsiding people. That's what really started the process of me connecting with other workers. There were a couple people I had reached out to, and we started chatting in Facebook Messenger. Then we created a little group—it was just the three of us—where we would have discussions and share information. The others told me about how the pay change was affecting them. What the change essentially did was it took away the transparency that we had previously had with our pay. Before, we could actually see what the formula was for how our pay was calculated. This change took that away from us, basically leaving us in the dark and switching to a non-transparent pay model, which we call a "blackbox algorithm." The algorithm determines our pay. It's run by artificial intelligence, and Shipt will not disclose to us how it works, other than saying it uses certain "variables" to calculate our pay. Personally, I find it hard to trust this algorithm when I already know that the technology Shipt and Target use can't even keep good track of what's in and out of stock at the stores (remember, Target owns Shipt). If they don't know what's in stock and what isn't, how are they going to understand how many people were in line on a particular day, at a particular time, and then calculate my pay accordingly? The more I learned about these "variables," the more I started to think, "Hey, this isn't good." Being the person that I am, asking questions the way that I do, I wanted to learn more—and the more that I learned, the more it drew me to other people.

Over the course of a two-week period—between January 20 and the first week of February—I spoke to over six hundred people. The last count I remember was 654 people—I lost count after that. I had conversations with people from all walks of life. I talked to single moms, I talked to husband-and-wife teams, I talked to college kids, bartenders, and all sorts of folks. The stories they told me were so powerful and so intriguing, because there was certainly a commonality between them, which was: "Hey, Shipt hit me with this pay cut and it's basically ruined me financially." People were telling me about how badly it impacted them, and about not knowing how they were going to pay their rent, how they were going to pay their mortgage, how they were going to pay their grocery bills, how they were going to pay for the basic necessities of life. Some people did say that they were doing this work to earn extra money for a vacation and things like that, but the majority of people relied on this income to live, because that's how Shipt sells it to you. Even to this day, they sell it as, "This is your little independent business; this is how you can make your business succeed." All of these people had bought into that—and, in a sense, I had too. At the beginning, when you're starting out, you believe that this is your thing, that you have all the power to control your earning potential. Then, in the middle of the night, without any warning, Shipt drops these changes and you see how little control you actually have. And so, hearing these stories from other shoppers was really impactful; that's what really led us to decide that somebody needed to speak up about this, and somebody needed to do something about it.

Max: So, obviously, I'm biased about this. We're having this conversation for a book of interviews with workers, so I think anyone will be able to tell right off the bat that I really believe in the power of workers sharing their stories with one another. But just hearing you talk about this now . . . it really reminded me of where that belief came from. My family basically lost everything in the Great Recession. My dad was a realtor and my mom was an interior designer, so both of their careers were tied to the housing market, which bottomed out in 2008. And for all the talk of an "economic recovery" in the years after that, things really only got worse for us and a lot of other families. My folks were looking everywhere for help but couldn't really find any. Then, eventually, we lost the house I grew up in. It was after that happened that my mom and dad started driving for Uber and Lyft.

My dad was never a really talkative guy, you know? I love my dad—he's a very funny, loving, quirky guy, but he was never a big chatterbox. That obviously got a lot worse after the recession. I could just tell that he was punishing himself inside, that he was blaming himself—as if the destructive force of a global economic recession was somehow all his personal fault. No matter how much I, my siblings, or my mom tried to convince him otherwise, it was almost impossible for him to hear that and take it to heart. I'll never forget the gradual change I could see in my dad, though, once he started driving for Uber just to pay the bills. He started getting into conversations with the passengers he was driving all over Southern California, and he realized that he was driving people who were his age to their second or third job, people who had immigrated to this country, like he did, and who had also lost their homes and all their savings in the recession. It was in that space, in his car, doing gig work, that my dad was finally able to talk to other workers about what they were going through, and he allowed himself to open up a bit more about what we had gone through. I think it took that experience for him to finally realize that it wasn't all his fault, that this was something affecting *a lot* of other people. And, I just . . . I've never forgotten how powerful that was, how much I could see the change in him. That's why I wanted to ask what it was like for you to talk to over six hundred people about this kind of thing. I imagine that you must have had a similar experience over the course of these conversations, some sort of dawning realization like, "Man, I'm not alone . . . this is happening to a lot of people."

Willy: Yeah. One of the problems I always run into is I can never do justice to these stories. You can never really convey the power of those moments when other workers are sharing their personal stories with you. And all of those conversations I had—it all began with one person, the first person I talked to. To this day, I still remember that conversation: It was with a single mom. I still don't really know why she decided to open up to me, a perfect stranger on Facebook. I just sent her a message like, "Hey, can you tell me about the pay change and how it's affected you?" and she just responded like, "Oh, let me tell you . . ." I opened up a can of worms there. She actually didn't live too far away from me—she lived in San Antonio, which is about a five-hour drive away from Dallas. So, it felt really close to home. And just having that conversation with her . . . it really affected me. She told me her story: that she was a single mom, that she had recently gotten out of an abusive relationship, that the low bar for entry was one of the main reasons she joined Shipt. She told me that she had been working for Shipt for about two and a half years, and that she really felt like she had found her home. She was really happy, her child was happy, everybody was happy. She was doing well for herself, she finally felt like she was starting to get out of the situation the bad relationship had left her in. When the changes to the pay structure hit her, she said that it took her back to the last day that she was in that abusive relationship with her significant other, that she felt as hopeless as she did the night before she decided to leave. She told me that she was able to leave because she had savings; now, that was not the case. With the pay changing the way it did, some people were reporting 30, 40, even 50 percent pay decreases. In the two weeks since the rollout of these changes, the woman told me her income had dropped by about 45 percent. That was a significant drop in pay for her, and she didn't know how she was going to provide for herself and her child. She teared up and started crying, and she told me, "I really don't know what to do—I feel helpless. I don't have any assistance or support, and Shipt won't even talk to me about this. All they've done is send me a canned email saying this is supposed to be better for me. A 45 percent pay cut is not better for me. You can't convince me otherwise. Now I'm sitting here struggling to figure out a way to make ends meet and to feed my child and myself."

That conversation really took me back to my upbringing. It made me remember the struggles my parents had trying to provide the basic necessities for us. I grew up in Texas, which is a conservative state, and my family is very conservative too—has been for many, many years. I've always been the type of person who will figure out a way to make something work. I'll strap my boots on, get to work, and figure it out. If it doesn't work out, then you just have to find another way. That's just the way I was raised. We were never looking for handouts, and we always tried to avoid putting ourselves in situations where we would have to resort to using food stamps or go on welfare or anything like that. But talking to other Shipt shoppers, seeing people struggling with making ends meet, it kind of took me back to the moment when my mom and dad were looking at each other and saying, "At this point, we're going to have to ask for assistance from the government just to feed our kids." Not to get too much into my mom and dad's relationship—they didn't end up staying together. My dad left and left my mom alone. So, there she was with four boys to feed, clothe, and take care of, and it looked like a really dire situation. Hearing this lady's story about Shipt and the situation she found herself in—it really took me right back to where my mom was and how much she had to struggle to raise us. That was my moment, that was when I decided this couldn't just go on. Somebody had to do something, and we were going to have to work together to make something happen.

I was never able to get back in contact with that first woman I talked to. I reached out to her a couple times afterward but never heard back. But all the conversations I had with workers after that, all the stories that I heard, that was all inspired by that first phone call. I wouldn't have been able to reach out to other shoppers, and we wouldn't have collectively come together to hear one another's stories, if it wasn't for her being strong enough to share her story with me. Everyone gets into organizing for different reasons. For me, the conversation that she and I had is what pushed me to reach out to people and invite them into this worker-led organizing we ended up creating with other Shipt shoppers. We called our group on Facebook "The SHIpT List."

But these stories aren't particular to one person or one type of family. Conservative, liberal, it doesn't matter. You can be whatever color, you can be whatever religion you want to be, and it still impacts you—it transcends politics, it transcends social status. These companies literally did this to people overnight. And they understand what they're doing, they know these pay changes are going to impact people's lives, and they don't care. Through these conversations that we had with other Shipt shoppers, we were able to identify what this pay change actually was, and we were able to see clearly that it was not good for workers. We continue to get reports from workers of their pay being dramatically lower than what Shipt said it was going to be.

Max: That's such an incredible story, man. Like you said, it's amazing how entire movements can grow out of the smallest interactions or the most random accidents. You find yourself in this situation, one thing kind of leads to another, and you just don't know where it's gonna go. It's amazing that someone like yourself, who was just looking for answers, ended up connecting with this other worker, whom you had never met, and having a conversation that would kickstart this whole collective process that is way bigger than any one shopper or any one app. And, I mean, it's such a Herculean task to make those connections in the first place, and to break yourself and others out of that pull-myself-up-by-my-bootstraps mentality. Having been very much sold on that mentality for a good chunk of my life, I know that it must have taken a whole lot of work to get people to break free of that.

It really makes me wonder what takeaway lessons there might be here, not just for other gig workers but for the labor movement writ large. Do you think this sets an example for folks around the country who are trying to connect with their coworkers and organize their workplace? And since we both grew up conservative, I can't help but ask: Do you think your conservative upbringing has helped you in any way with your organizing? Do you think it helps you connect with people—especially people who have that rugged individualist, bootstrap mentality—to be able to speak to those conservative values like self-sufficiency, personal responsibility, dignity, and pride? Those aren't exclusively conservative values, of course, but you get what I mean . . .

Willy: I would say so, yes. I think having been raised conservative, and having had that viewpoint for so many years, really has empowered me to see this from a different perspective than the majority of people I've talked to. I think that what the labor movement as a whole can take away from our story is that you can't generalize people into these big buckets and categories. Each individual person you interact with is a human being with a story, and every single story is extremely valuable.

I understand different viewpoints and I respect them 100 percent, but I think the conversations that happen on the conservative side tend to revolve around this idea that if you don't like it, you should just go get another job. I hear that all the time. People will say, "Okay, you're a Shipt shopper and you guys have these grievances, but no one's really doing anything about it. Just go find another job." That's not the right way to handle things. I used to have that mentality. I used to think, "Well, why are you still in that bad situation? Why are you still climbing that tree if you know you're about to fall?" When I'm having these conversations with people, having that perspective as a former conservative has really given me the ability to listen to the actual heart of the story. It helps me think, "What is it that drives that person to be who they are and find themselves in the situation they're in? How can they find their way out of it? And, more importantly, how can we collectively work together to find solutions to these problems?" That's really helped me be able to connect with people, to look past their socio-economic status or whatever, and to try to find a solution. This work was sold to them as a business venture. They thought they were buying into and building their own independent business, and now they find themselves beholden to and dependent on the big businesses of the gig economy. Basically, they were lied to—it was a bait-and-switch, and more control was exerted upon them than they realized. The mindset I grew up with would tell me: If you find yourself in that situation, the only way out is to buckle down even more and pull yourself out of this rut. But after having had so many conversations with other workers and even some very liberal friends of mine—at this point, I call them friends, because they are my friends—I've grown out of that mindset. I've realized that to go up against a multibillion-dollar corporation, you need to have collective action. That's not what my dad taught me, you know? "You go and you fight your battles alone, son"—those are the kinds of conversations we had when I was growing up. But if I tried to take on Target or Shipt by myself, they would completely destroy me in a matter of a day—in a matter of hours, actually, if they really wanted to. It takes collective action and a tremendous amount of people working together in unison to get your voices out there and to get people to listen to what you're saying.

The fact is: nobody cares about your condition more than you. But if you can put your story out there, what you say may resonate with other people. Their ears might perk up. They might say, "Hey, that happened to me at my job," or, "I'm in a similar financial situation," and then they actually listen. That might help them start to see the larger inequities that are being created by these companies. They'll start to see the bigger picture beyond their own sphere, which is what companies like Shipt don't want to happen. That's the direction we've been going in, and that's allowed us to take the conversation to a level where people will actually listen to us. And I think it's really important that we've gotten to that point, and that we've done it in a way that is not about one singular person or one group of people. Because this is definitely not about me or any other individual gig worker; it's about all of us, as a gig-worker community. The problem now is that we are struggling to get the rest of the country to listen to us and to hear conversations about the gig economy from the perspective of gig workers ourselves. And gig companies are doing everything they can to drown out our voices. Just the other day, for instance, I heard an interview with Dara Khosrowshahi, the CEO of Uber, and he was talking about Proposition 22[6] and everything that happened with that campaign

---

6 Proposition 22 was a ballot initiative in the state of California that passed with 59 percent of the vote in November 2020. After the passing of Assembly Bill 5 in September 2019, which extended the designation of employee (and the full suite of labor protections that come with that designation) to most wage-earning workers in California, app-based companies like Uber, Lyft, DoorDash, and PostMates pooled their resources and collectively spent over $200 million in an effort to have themselves exempted from AB5 by way of a ballot measure that would be decided by voters. As of today, the jaw-dropping amount of money spent by these tech companies has made Prop 22 the most expensive ballot measure in California history. Moreover, in an unheard-of move, the authors of Prop 22 also included language in the ballot measure that would make it virtually impossible to amend, stipulating that a seven-eighths supermajority of the Legislature would be required to do so. With the passage of Prop 22, gig workers in California continued to be classified as "independent contractors," which negates their right to basic protections and benefits like overtime pay, unemployment insurance, family and sick leave, personal protective equipment provided by companies during the COVID-19 pandemic, the right to unionize, etc.

in California. He said that, prior to Prop 22, Uber had been reaching out to labor unions so they could have conversations among themselves about "third way" solutions for gig workers. Did they reach out to us, though? Look, I respect unions and any ally that wants to fight with us, but *we* are the ones who are aggrieved. And unions cannot unionize us anyway. We can't even unionize ourselves—it's not possible in the gig economy because of our legal status. If we did, it wouldn't be recognized by the National Labor Relations Board. There was no real reason for Uber to even go to these unions other than to try to game the system in their favor or, at best, to just make it appear like they cared about workers. The conversation needs to be with the gig workers ourselves, not with people outside the gig economy who cannot represent us or even share in the reasons why we're aggrieved. Yes, there are some basic protections and borderline things that can be addressed by people and groups outside of this community. But the fact of the matter is: We're the ones who are aggrieved, we're the ones putting our vehicles and our lives on the line every single day to make the gig economy function, and we're the ones who should be driving the discussion. And that discussion transcends politics, it transcends liberal or conservative backgrounds—it's about the human experience, and it's about what that experience looks like when you do the work that gig workers do.

Max: Since you mentioned Proposition 22, I think it's important we talk about that for a second. It passed in November of 2020. The disinformation campaign behind it, the most expensive campaign for a single ballot measure in U.S. history—over $200 million, funded by gig companies like Uber, Lyft, and DoorDash—was just bombarding people in California for months, and the effects are going to be felt for years and decades to come. Prop 22 may very well mean that so many of the things you described, so many of the grievances gig workers deal with on a daily basis, are going to be the norm for the foreseeable future.

Update: On August 20, 2021, months after this interview was recorded, Superior Court Judge Frank Roesch in Alameda County, California, ruled that Proposition 22 was unconstitutional and unenforceable in response to a lawsuit brought forth by three rideshare drivers and the Service Employees International Union (SEIU). Gig companies like the ones that pushed for 22 will certainly appeal the ruling, and it remains to be seen what the final outcome will be.

If anything, from Donald Trump becoming president to COVID-19, these past few years have taught me to be exceedingly humble when it comes to making predictions about the future [laughs]. But I truly believe that, in decades to come, people will look back and see Prop 22 as a major turning point in labor history. It was the moment when the gig companies from Silicon Valley were able to take incredible amounts of money and incredible amounts of lies told to the voting public and use them to essentially brute force this ballot measure into reality, which has allowed those same companies to rewrite labor laws to fit their exploitative business model. Like you said, it has essentially solidified a permanent underclass of workers, a "third category" of workers who will legally be making a lot less than minimum wage and who will not get the kind of protections they deserve. And other states around the country have been taking notice, because if Prop 22 could pass in deep blue California, it can pass anywhere, right? I think what we're going to see in years to come is a lot of other states and a lot of other businesses trying to build on what gig companies accomplished with Prop 22. And I really, really worry that, bit by bit, more of the full-time and part-time work model will break apart, and the workforce of the future will become a free-floating army of underpaid, under-protected task rabbits. Prop 22 was a major advance in the class war that we've been living through, and I guess I worry we won't realize how destructive it is until it's way too late. But what do you think? What will Prop 22 mean for the future of work in this country? What will it mean for gig workers and organizers like yourself?

Willy: Personally, I don't view Prop 22 and what happened in California as the end-all-be-all of this story, nor do I think it will be the unchallenged law of the land forever. This was the most classic bait-and-switch that has ever been pulled off, and I think that the voting public, regulators, judicial branches, etc.—not just in the state of California, but the entire federal government—are quickly going to realize how much gig companies exploited them and gamed the system to get 22 passed. Over $200 million were spent on a disinformation campaign designed to trick the public into thinking that they were voting for a law that was supposedly going to be good for gig workers. These gig companies are really good at convincing people that whatever they're pushing, whatever measure they're taking—whether it be a pay cut, or Prop 22, or whatever—is going to be good for the worker and for society as a whole. Of course, this is the furthest thing from the truth, and I think Prop 22 is exposing that.

When 22 first came on my radar and I started to really understand what it was, why it was important, and how much it would take to fight against it, I felt very daunted—it seemed like an insurmountable task. I thought, "How in the heck is one guy and one group of ragtag shoppers going to take on 22?" But we quickly realized that one advantage we have is that we don't have to spend any money. Here we are going up against $200 million and we don't have anything . . . the large majority of the work we do is self-funded. We've taken a few donations here and there, but not much. And yet, we feel like our voices were very much part of the conversation about Prop 22. Not as much as we would have liked, of course, but we were still in the fight, we were still being heard, and it didn't cost us a penny.

I think that the effects of Prop 22 are going to show the nation and the voting public how much these companies really are exploiting gig workers, and that we need to put a stop to it. These companies are being given an extreme amount of power and control over supposedly "independent" contractors, but I think the thing that's really important for people to realize is that these companies have taken the route they've taken because they could not actually win in court. *That's* the biggest takeaway of Prop 22 for me. By the letter of the law, gig workers have actually been employees for a long time, and these gig companies could not successfully prove otherwise in the court system. Instead of going through the courts and winning their battles that way, and instead of going through the standard process of getting laws passed through the legislature—and, thus, ensuring that those laws didn't violate basic labor rights protected by the government—they went the "third route." They took the route that they know best: purchasing influence, buying their way to getting what they want. That's why they created this $200 million war chest, which they used to misinform the public. I saw some of the ads that were flying around in California. There were all these "voting guide" ads that said, "If you're progressive, vote this way," or, "If you're going to vote for Biden, vote 'Yes' on 22." Sadly, this misinformation campaign really did trick a lot of people.

But the most encouraging sign for me was what happened in San Francisco. These gig companies—Uber, Shipt, DoorDash, etc.—all have headquarters there, and it was pretty incredible to see that in their own backyard, 60 percent of the electorate overwhelmingly voted "No" on Prop 22. That's because gig workers have such a strong organizing foothold in San Francisco. Where we were strong, where we were able to have our voices heard, even though we were completely outmatched on spending, the general electorate recognized by a 60 to 40 percent margin that Prop 22 was bad. And so, while we may have lost the state, I think it goes to show the power of gig workers to collectively bring our voices together, to yell as loudly as we possibly can, and to have the public hear our cries. At the end of the day, it's not just the electorate who's watching, but regulators too. I know because they reach out to us. I've had interviews and really long conversations with a number of regulators. I can't disclose which ones, because those are ongoing investigations. These gig companies may think they're the only ones with a voice, but they're not. I don't think it should go unnoticed or unappreciated that we do have the power to draw attention to these issues and to shape these tough conversations. And they *are* tough conversations. For instance, the more I learn about Prop 22 and its effects, the more I can see how gig companies have deliberately put true independent contractors, or freelancers, in the center of the discussion and pitted them against gig workers. They've used AB-5—the California bill that Prop 22 was designed to overturn—to draw attention to problems freelancers face with their employment status, classification, and treatment by prospective employers. In so doing, they've invited a tremendous amount of hate from the freelancer community, which has been directed at the gig workers AB-5 protected. But the reality is that it's the gig companies, not the gig workers, who have created these problems—that's where the anger should be directed.

Here's the thing: The Prop 22 conversation, the AB-5 conversation—this all stems from the fact that gig companies have been exploiting the misclassification of workers since 2009, or thereabouts, up to today. They've created an untenable situation that benefits them and hurts society, and that really needs to be addressed. I think the pandemic has put that need front and center. When I have these conversations with regulators, that's usually what they're looking into. They're investigating the financial holes that the gig economy is putting states in. Workers, states, and society as a whole are being put in a really tough situation—we're the ones bearing the costs of the gig economy while these gig companies continue to increase their profitability margins. Throughout the pandemic, and throughout the Prop 22 campaign, it has been genuinely unsettling to watch top executives at companies like DoorDash enrich themselves and become billionaires. It's really infuriating to watch this happen because, from a gig worker perspective, I know that those companies are nothing without us. It's our vehicles and our effort that make those grocery deliveries or meal deliveries happen. We're the ones who make the gig economy run. Without us, these companies don't exist. But I think there's a reckoning coming for these companies. They've been exploiting misclassification this entire time. Their whole business model is based on it, and at some point they're going to have to answer for it.

5. Courtney Smith

My name is Courtney Smith. I live in Detroit, Michigan, and I am thirty-one years old. I am a full-time single parent, teacher, and organizer.

Max: Damn, I was actually living in Michigan for the past eight years. I was in Ann Arbor, though, a little down the road. Are you originally from Detroit?

Courtney: I am not. I moved to Detroit in the middle of the pandemic, in May. I'm originally from Des Moines, Iowa. I don't know if you know much about Iowa—I guess the only thing that we're really known for is, like, meth and corn [laughs] . . .

Max: [Laughs.] And the caucuses!

Courtney: And the Iowa caucuses! Every four years we get high energy from that. So, yeah, Iowa—that's where I was born and raised.

Max: Were you a corn girl?

Courtney: I was a corn girl. [Laughs.] Thank God.

Max: You know, truth be told, I think I've only been to Iowa once. And that's not a knock on Iowa, there just haven't been many occasions that have taken me there. So I have no real frame of reference for what it would be like to grow up there. Did you have a lot of family there?

Courtney: Yeah, my whole family is from Iowa. When people think of Iowa, a lot of them assume that you must be living on a farm surrounded by cornfields and whatnot. But I lived in the capital, Des Moines. It's a smaller city—less than a million people live there—but it's still pretty big in comparison to the rural towns. It's a small big city, I guess. I think it's similar to Detroit in that way, which is actually one of the things that drew me to Detroit: It's a city, but it still has that small-town community feeling. Unlike Detroit, though, there's not much to do in Des Moines. We don't have our own sports team, we don't have a whole lot of entertainment stuff going on. I guess that's why there's such a big meth industry in Iowa. Because, really, that's all there is to do there: go out to bars and . . . those sorts of things. Growing up in Iowa, though, I would say I had a typical childhood. I was playing in the streets with my friends and doing the sort of things that you see kids in bigger cities doing.

Max: So, paint me a picture here. When you were growing up in Iowa, playing in the street and all that, were y'all playing sports, or jump rope, or what? I guess I always feel a little guilty about this kind of thing because, having grown up in Southern California, we have the exact opposite problem over there. If you're a kid in Southern California it can be pretty great, because there's just *so* much stuff . . .

Courtney: Right, right.

Max: Southern California is one of those rare places where you could drive an hour in any direction and end up at either the beach, the desert, or the mountains—that's pretty special. But on top of all that, you obviously have all the malls, all the promenades, you have Disneyland and a bunch of other theme parks, you have a lot of sports teams, you have Hollywood . . . honestly, it's almost like a constant sensory overload when you're growing up there. But we still made a lot of our own fun. My brothers, friends, and I would make treehouses, ride our bikes around, go on little adventures, all that good stuff. For kids like you in Iowa, though, I imagine you must have gotten really good at making your own fun [laughs].

Courtney: Yeah, we definitely got good at that, because we didn't have any of those things you're talking about, really. It's funny because when *we* say we're "going to the beach," we're talking about going to this man-made lake that's dirty and gross. You can't see through the water, most people don't want to swim in it. We grew up poor, though, so we had to find a lot of free activities to do. We had no qualms about going to swim in this dirty-ass lake [laughs]. That was our fun. We loved being outdoors as kids. It was nothing like what you see today with so many kids stuck in their houses and just playing video games and watching TV. We didn't even have cable growing up, at least not until I was in my teenage years. I have a lot of siblings—I'm the third oldest of seven—so I had them to keep me occupied and play around with. We would sumo wrestle, for instance. We would put pillows underneath our shirts and then charge at each other as fast as we could.

Max: [Laughs.] Yes! We did that too!

Courtney: We would play-fight outside. I got into a lot of fights growing up [laughs].

Max: [Laughs.] Technically, you could also count that as a form of entertainment . . .

Courtney: Yes, exactly. It can definitely be its own form of entertainment. We also went sledding almost every single day it snowed. It snows a lot in Des Moines, so we had that to keep us occupied during the winter. We had snowball fights, built snowmen, and all that fun stuff that you only see in movies now.

Max: That was something I was always very jealous of growing up—I always wanted it to snow. I used to fantasize about having a white Christmas. We were lucky if it got below sixty degrees around Christmas. And I fully realize, especially now that I've spent many years living in the Midwest, that I'm not going to get a whole lot of sympathy from people when I say that.

Courtney: [Laughs.] No, not at all. It's funny, too, because every time it snows now my son thinks that it's Christmas . . .

Max: Aww, that's really sweet.

Courtney: Yeah. We just had a snowstorm and he came running to me like, "Is it Christmas? Is Santa coming again?" I had to tell him, "Oh, no, Santa's not coming right now . . ."

Max: [Laughs.] "Santa is gonna go broke!"

Courtney: [Laughs.] Exactly.

Max: Man, it's funny how you make those sorts of connections as a kid, though. It reminds me of how, growing up in a place where it's hot and sunny like 90 percent of the year, the thing that was most exciting for us was when it would rain. It was like an event. My siblings and I would get all excited and go out and play in the rain, we would go exploring and wear our little jackets—it was a blast. But the thing that most sticks out in my mind is: Whenever it would rain, my mom would make hot chocolate and soup . . . and my mom makes the best soups. That was the best part about rainy days—for me, at least. I remember when El Niño happened in the '90s and it was raining all the time, I got really fat from all the soup and hot chocolate [laughs]. That was one of the best times of my childhood, now that I think about it. I'm getting all nostalgic now . . .

Speaking of nostalgia, I was cracking up when you were talking about growing up in Iowa and you said that "going to the beach" for you guys meant swimming in this dirty-ass, man-made lake. So, I *may* have oversold Southern California a bit [laughs]. Yeah, the beach is great, the mountains are great, the desert is great, but in-between all of that you've just got this endless sprawl. When you're flying into LAX you can see it: From the mountains to the ocean, it's just freeways and houses and buildings and grid as far as the eye can see. Where we lived—around the Anaheim, Orange County, area—the only real lakes you could go to were these big, rectangular, man-made lakes off the freeway. I still have great memories of those lakes, though, because my dad, who loves to fish, would always take us out there. "Going fishing" for us meant sleeping in the car, then waking up around four in the morning when my dad would be driving through the entrance of one of these big man-made lakes. And the funniest part about it is my dad would say things to us like, "You guys see that big, industrial drainage pipe where all the water's coming out? That's the sweet spot—that's where all the good fish are." [Laughs.] It may not have been the most idyllic fishing setting, but we had fun.

Courtney: There's a lot of those little things in my childhood that I didn't really pick up on at the time, but now that I have this, I guess you could say, more anti-capitalist critique of the world, I notice things that I hadn't noticed before. It kind of provides you with, like, a new layer of experience on top of everything. So, hearing about this industrial pipe draining into the lake, I'm imagining there's probably a bunch of debris and pollution in that lake as well, right? But you don't think about that when you're little. Having that way of understanding the world kind of adds a more interesting layer over your life, and it kind of clears out the muck—at least it has for me. I don't know if you've had the same experience.

Max: Oh, I definitely have. Honestly, a lot of that perspective has come from having the kind of conversations we're having now, and I'm really grateful for that. I think that's one of the reasons I appreciate these conversations so much. It feels like you're working out that perspective together, like each person is bringing what they have to the conversation . . . thoughts, memories, etc. Then you put that stuff together, you learn from each other, and you help each other shape that larger perspective, if that makes sense.

Actually, now that I think of it, that's why I started my podcast, *Working People*, in the first place. That whole project started with me interviewing my dad a few years after we had lost everything in the Great Recession. My dad is Mexican by birth. He became a citizen in the 1980s. He was born into poverty and he had a rough childhood. He didn't really grow up having the kind of emotional tools to talk about trauma or anything like that. There was a lot of stuff in his own past, including all the shit our family went through in the recession, that he just couldn't process—none of us were able to process it, really. We weren't talking to each other about it. We were just kind of receding further into ourselves, punishing ourselves, lamenting all that we had lost. Because that's what you do when you don't have the perspective you're talking about, right? If you don't have a larger frame of reference to understand how the economy and politics work, and how they can both be so cruel to working people, you just accept that cruelty as, like, the natural order of things. And you internalize it too. If you don't see how much the system is rigged against you, then whenever you struggle to get ahead in that system you take it as a deeply personal failure. Anyway, that's why I started doing these sorts of interviews with workers, because I saw that when I gave my dad the chance to just tell his story and talk openly for as long as he wanted to, it finally let him work through some stuff, and it let us work through that stuff together. We were able to talk about what our family had been through, and talking about it was what helped us gain that perspective. Now, after having so many conversations over the years like that one, and this one, I'm able to reflect on the world in a really different way. Like you said, even when I'm reflecting on little things, like memories from my childhood, I can see them in a new light now. I still really cherish those memories, of course. But it does add that extra layer, like you were saying. Now, the deeper I look into why all the fish were congregating around that big, industrial pipe, the less romantic the story gets [laughs].

Courtney: Oh, no! I didn't mean to minimize the romanticism in your story. I was just saying that perspective adds something that wasn't there before. For me, growing up poor, no one in my family really valued education—me and my sister were the first to go on to college. Well, I shouldn't say they didn't "value" it; it's more that they didn't have time for it. They had to work all the time, and when you're just trying to survive it's hard to think about other things. And so, before I got that education, I didn't understand the ways that the government and the economy impacted my life. Now, when I reflect on my childhood, or when I hear someone else's story, I pick up on those things a little bit more. It's like my sensors are on. Now, when people are talking, those sensors will go off like, "*Beep*, that's capitalism!" or, "*Beep*, that's a local policy decision!" You know what I mean? You see the outside forces that have fucked up their lives, or your own life. It doesn't make those stories from our past any less romantic. I think it makes it more nuanced and interesting.

Max: I think you're totally right, and I really loved the way that you put that. It's a hard thing to put into words, but it's like: When you're a kid, you're more able to have this sense that the world is just *out there*, that it's this big, open thing, and that you're just moving through it, right? As an adult, though, you start to see more of the ways that the world leaves its mark on you—how it limits you, how it directs you, how it shapes you. You no longer see yourself as this kind of free-floating human being in a big, open world. You see yourself more as this person who often can't live the life you want because the world is pushing you in certain directions, taking away certain opportunities, bogging you down with bills and credit scores and whatever. The world gets more rigid and suffocating as you get older. And it's sad that we just call that dealing with the "responsibilities" of adulthood or whatever. Because a lot of that *is* the result of government policies, it's the result of how the economy is set up, etc. And the more you see and understand that, like you said, the more you get this nuanced and textured understanding of the world that you're a part of, and that's definitely not a bad thing.

Courtney: Oh, yeah! I've honestly found it to be more empowering, because I think the conversations we have in this country are so individualized and atomized. It's all "competition" this and "self-help" that, and it all just amounts to telling the individual that it's all up to you for your life to be a certain way. That's why I don't think people really understand how they are impacted by their environment. I know I certainly didn't. And that was especially hard when I got sober—there was a lot of self-hate and blame there. Once I finally did come to that understanding, it was like an awakening . . . I realized it wasn't all my fault. I started to look at my life and see, "Oh, this thing was a barrier," or, "I didn't have access to this kind of service, which would have helped me get through this situation." Those sorts of things started to help me realize that I'm not all to blame here. No matter how many self-help books I devoured, no matter how much I went to therapy and took all the classes that I could find, at the end of the day capitalism is still a barrier. It's always going to be the thing telling you, "You're not enough." And so, I finally got to a point where I was like, "You know what? Fuck that. I *am* enough, and I'm done changing myself. Now it's time to change the system." For me, having that perspective provided a real sense of empowerment—and it was healing too, in a way, because I knew it wasn't all my fault.

Max: Wow, that's really, really powerful, and I thought you put that so beautifully. And, like you said, it's not just relevant to your own story.

Coming to that realization is *such* a big step for so many of us—and, sadly, a lot of people never take that step, because we live in a society that encourages us to see everything as our fault. If you're feeling like shit because your boss, or your landlord, or whoever is treating you like shit, it's 100 percent your problem and your responsibility to fix. And if you can't fix it, if you don't feel better, that's your fault too. This is where that whole pull-yourself-up-by-your-bootstraps stuff comes from . . .

Courtney: There ya go! That's what I was trying to think of. The words were right there at the tip of my tongue but I couldn't remember . . .

Max: It's part of the same illusion, right? It's this illusion that you're raised with in the U.S. that any success you hope to have, any dream you want to achieve, is entirely within your control—you've just gotta work hard enough to get it. And if you don't get it, you didn't work hard enough. To be able to finally say "This isn't entirely my fault" is such a huge shift from how we're trained to see ourselves. I've seen and experienced that firsthand. That was the kind of shift that me, my dad, and our family went through, and it took a long time to get there. It took almost a decade to get my parents to realize that a global recession was not entirely their fault.

Courtney: Yeah, I can't imagine going through that. You still hear about the recession and everything that happened, but you never hear the stories of the individuals and what they went through, the feelings that they must have felt. The anxiety of not being able to keep up with your mortgage, the pain and fear of the sheriff coming to your home and removing your belongings or, you know, however that situation plays out . . . I've been evicted before, so I know the shame that comes with it. I know the barriers that you have to face afterward when you're trying to get housing, and all the ways the government has astronomically failed people in that position. So, yeah, I can't imagine what your family must have gone through during that time . . .

Max: Well, you were talking a little bit about this yourself earlier. When you were describing the long, arduous journey you had to go through to finally see the world the way you see it now, to see how your environment impacted you. If you're okay discussing it, could we talk about that environment? You mentioned a few things, like how your folks were always working and how you and your sister were the first to go to college, or to even feel like college was an option.

Courtney: So, I'm biracial: My mom is White, my dad's Black. When my mom got pregnant with my older brother—she was sixteen—she knew that her parents weren't going to be okay with it, because she was pregnant by a Black man. She was worried that they were going to force her to get an abortion, because they did the same thing to her sister when she got pregnant by a Black man. My grandma's response was, "What are you going to do with a biracial child?" And this is, like, in the '80s, so it wasn't like it was super uncommon . . . interracial marriages were legal and whatnot. So my mom ended up leaving home, she dropped out of high school and had my brother when she was seventeen, and then had me and my twin sister when she was nineteen. By the time she was twenty-two, I believe, she had four kids. Just imagine being a single mom with no high-school education having four children, all in diapers. My mother really struggled to raise us. And along with that came other catastrophic things she experienced. Her sister had committed suicide when we were younger, so she kind of went through a really deep, dark depression during that time and couldn't keep a job. She started using drugs. The only thing that really saved us during that time was that we lived in public housing, which was income-based. Whenever she would lose a job, our rent would go down to like twenty bucks or something manageable. I don't really have full memories of these things—they've kind of been filled in by what my mom has told us now. But there were times in our lives when we didn't have furniture in the house. There were times when we would have to eat peanut butter and jelly for a month, because she couldn't get food stamps until the next month. Things like that.

My dad came back from the army with a drinking problem and an anger problem, and he ended up getting a felony assault charge, which then prevented him from being able to get jobs. He started relying on the underground economy to survive. A little caveat here: I used to be really ashamed to say that my father was a drug dealer—until I moved to

Michigan. I was at dinner with some friends and this White guy was just talking loudly about how his pot business was thriving, and I was like, "Wow. My whole life I was so ashamed that my dad was a drug dealer. Now it's legal in Michigan and my father still can't get a job." Where's the justice in that? I've seen him struggle my whole life. And, for obvious reasons, that caused him to have more brushes with the law. My dad was in and out of prison for a lot of my life. So I kind of had a real, visceral . . . I don't know if it was hatred for cops . . . it was just a deep fear of cops, because they would take away my dad.

Growing up with all of that created some of my own trauma. Luckily, I was able to graduate high school. My parents weren't able to do extra stuff to help us get through school. They couldn't really help with our homework, they didn't really stay on top of us to make sure we were doing our homework. It was just like a "Make sure you get it done," or "Make sure you're getting good grades" kind of thing. Because they were struggling so hard to survive and to just get through life, their involvement was very hands-off, I guess. They would try to do things like get us into extracurricular activities, but we couldn't afford it—we would start something and then end up having to quit two months later when they asked for more money. So, I was never really able to get into those things that would keep me busy and, you know, keep me out of trouble. Because of all the trauma that I experienced as a child, and the trauma of just being poor, I started drinking at a really young age. I think the first time I had a drink was when I was eleven, and it kind of just progressed from there. Obviously, I didn't start off a full-blown alcoholic, but by the time I was twenty-one I had a full-blown addiction. I still managed to get through high school, went on to college, and that's when things started getting out of control for me. I ended up dropping out of college, got into this abusive relationship, and became pregnant with my son. I had my son when I was twenty-three and . . . he's just been the light of my life. When I had my son, I realized that I didn't want him to go through the same things that I went through growing up. So I left. I left my abusive relationship and everything that I knew, I checked myself into a treatment facility, and I started the journey of getting sober and healing from all of the things that I had experienced growing up. And that was actually the year that Trump was elected . . .

Max: Oh, God! Don't tell me we're gonna pile Trump on top of everything?

Courtney: [Laughs.] Yeah! So, um, my whole worldview was blown up when Trump was elected. Because I found out that my mom had actually voted for Trump, and I was like, "What? How the fuck could you do this? This man is clearly racist, he's a homophobe, he's all these terrible things. And here you are with five mixed-race children and a Mexican husband! And you vote for Trump?" Mind you, she had voted for Obama both times before—she'd voted Democrat her entire life up until that point. I was really confused, and I couldn't accept the narrative that everybody who voted for Trump was racist. Because I know my mom. I know that she loves us with every particle of her being. I mean, she spent her entire life raising her children, doing the best she could for us, and sacrificing everything for us. For me, that wasn't an answer that I was willing to accept. I wanted to really understand how this could happen, how Trump could get elected, and what it meant for the country. Because I also didn't want to buy into the liberal hysteria of it all, like, "Oh, my God! Trump's gonna ruin everything!" Remember, at that point in my life, I was in a treatment facility living off of $300 a month for a good year. I was *poor* poor. We're talking, like, penny pinching just trying to eat, scraping up any resource or help that I could get to provide for me and my son. I was using cash assistance benefits—that's where the $300 a month came from. Things were *already* bad for me. And I think that's something that's typically left out of the story we tell ourselves about Donald Trump. When people talk about how terrible Trump was, they forget that things were already pretty bad for poor people in this country. The hysteria around Trump made me really curious about what was really happening, and the amount of people who voted for him was obviously dumbfounding.

Long story short, I decided to go back to school to get my degree. I wanted to become a social studies teacher, so I was studying history, economics, government, psychology, sociology, and I was really trying to understand how these systems that govern us affect us on an individual level—going from macro all the way to the micro. And I learned a lot. I should say that that's when I was first even introduced to the word "capitalism," to be honest. I did not grow up with an understanding of the economy or politics at all. All you would really hear, I guess, was that the

Republicans are for businesses and the business side of things, and the Democrats are more about cultural representation and that sort of thing. Being biracial and poor, I didn't feel like either party really touched on my actual, concrete world. It wasn't until I started learning about capitalism and how it affected me on an individual level that I really started to see through the fog of this whole "Republicans vs. Democrats" WrestleMania thing they got going on.

At the same time that I was going to school, I decided I wanted to give back to my community, so I started working for an after-school organization in the public schools there, teaching kids how to read, write, and perform poetry.

Max: That's awesome.

Courtney: Yeah, it was my favorite job ever. I loved the impact that it had on kids and the outlet that it gave them. It gave me a good outlet too. For me, it was a tool to cope and heal. I put everything I had into that job, and I worked my way up to being the director of the program. When I got the promotion, though, they had me fill out some paperwork that asked if I had ever been convicted of anything. So I checked "Yes" because I have an assault charge on my record, which had been expunged at that point. I had been there for two years already, and I had told them when they hired me in the first place that I had this charge, so I didn't think anything of it when I marked the box. Then they ended up emailing me, asking for more information, and digging deeper into it. They actually pulled the police arrest record of the incident. In the end, they basically told me that I was too violent to be working with kids, that it hadn't been long enough since the incident for me to be rehabilitated, and that I was no longer hirable. This was 2018, but the charge that they were looking into happened in 2012, so there was a good six-year gap in which I had gone through my probation and been rehabilitated. I had done all of these things I needed to do, and I had really turned my life around. For them to tell me that it was not long enough for me to be rehabilitated and that I no longer had a job, which was how I was feeding myself and my son, it was absolutely devastating.

I tried fighting it: I wrote letters; all the students, parents of students, and teachers I had worked with wrote letters on my behalf. I had the assistant superintendent, my bosses, everybody fighting on my behalf. But they were like, "Nope. Because you had already admitted guilt, it doesn't matter that the charge was expunged." And because it was a "right to work" state with at-will employment, they can technically do that. They can fire you for any reason they want, really, and they just found a good one. So they fired me, and it shattered the entire plan that I thought I had for my life, because this was the same school district that I planned to teach in once I finished my degree. I was . . . paralyzed. "What am I going to do now?" Then the shame sets in, you know? You start telling yourself, "It's my fault. I shouldn't have done this thing so many years ago. My past is still haunting me, and I can never run from it." After you kind of get over the shame, then you become angry. Then you start thinking, "Wait, is there no such thing as redemption? If we're not going to allow people the chance to turn their lives around and show that they're better human beings who can function in society, then what is the whole point of the criminal justice system?"

It was around that time that I ended up going to a Bernie Sanders rally. That was the first time in my life that I had ever heard a politician who talked about real problems that I had faced in my life, and who provided policy solutions that would actually make my life better. I remember the first rally that I went to, I cried. I cried while I was there, because I was so touched and . . . sorry, I'm tearing up now . . . it was the first time that I realized it wasn't all my fault. It was the first time I realized that I deserve better, and that I should demand better. And so, at that point, I started volunteering for the Bernie campaign. They had a campaign strategy to hire people who came from the communities they were organizing in, so when they told me they were hiring I applied immediately, got the job, and started working for Bernie Sanders. I started organizing for the first time ever, with no political background whatsoever. I never in my life thought I would ever go into politics. I absolutely despise politics—even now, even though I'm an organizer, I still fucking hate it [laughs]. But I know that it will make a difference. Also, I've found organizing to be a good way to, like, cope with capitalism and all that comes with it.

One more detail to add to this story, which brings us to now, to the COVID-19 pandemic: A week after I was hired by the Bernie campaign my older brother committed suicide. He had struggled his entire life with addiction and schizophrenia, and he had multiple suicide attempts in the past. So . . . I don't know if I can adequately explain the complicated feelings that come along with that. When you kind of know . . . I don't want to say we expected it, but it was like, because he had tried so many times before, we kind of always thought that that was the way he would probably die. Six months before his last attempt, he had tried again and ended up in the hospital. He had taken a bunch of pills and he had to be restrained, so there was a police officer there. I guess when they restrained him he assaulted the police officer. They ended up letting him go from the hospital. They didn't give him any follow-up care, no plan or anything—just sent him on his way, but then they pressed charges on him. I think his life just kind of spiraled after that. And so, when it finally happened, I was just in shock. And I was concerned, too, because I was used to working jobs where you can't take time off, you can't be sick, etc. Working for Bernie's campaign was the first time I had a "real job" that gave me benefits and actually cared about my wellbeing. It's really sad to say, honestly, but my first thought was, "I'm going to get fired. This is it." Luckily, that didn't happen—they gave me some time off to deal, to grieve. Then, when I went back two weeks later, I really hammered down and got to work. I think the whole experience gave me more of a sense of urgency about why we so desperately need policies like Medicare for All, criminal justice reform, housing for all, and things like that. Because I had seen the way that my brother had been impacted by all of those things, or the lack of those things. So, I don't know, if we lived in a world where Bernie Sanders had been elected in 2016, my brother might still be here . . .

Max: My God . . . I'm so sorry, Courtney. You know, I'm thinking about what you said earlier about yourself, about your long path out of addiction and how important it was to recognize and come to terms with the fact that the world does shape who we are, that our environment does have an impact on us. Sometimes our environments really hurt us, and this fucking society just doesn't care enough about its people to treat that pain, let alone prevent it. I can hear that pain in your story—and I thank you so much for being open about it and sharing it with me. I can't imagine all that pain that you and your family have gone through.

One thing that really struck me was how many parts of your story are recognizable to me. Just to give one example: I'm mixed race. My dad's Mexican, my mom's White . . . well, she's part Mexican, part Italian, but for all intents and purposes she's a White lady. So, my siblings and I all grew up mixed race, and we grew up pretty conservative too. And my dad—again, a Mexican immigrant who had grown up dirt poor in Tijuana, and who had lost everything in the recession—voted for Donald Trump.

Courtney: Wow.

Max: That's why I was so struck by what you said about your mom: how you couldn't accept the predominant narrative in 2016 that people were using to try to explain away how Donald Trump could get elected. Because, like you said—I thought you put this perfectly before—when Trump got elected, everyone was looking for reasons to explain it that *didn't* implicate themselves. It was much easier to paint Trump as a monstrous outlier than to take a hard look at the system that had not only created Trump, but that had also created so much misery, so much pain, so much disaffection and resentment, and so much unfairness that it drove enough people to be attracted to someone like Trump. And that was the case for my dad. Just like you, I wouldn't accept the lazy narrative that the only problem was that people like your mom are just racist and that's why they voted for Trump. I couldn't accept the same explanation when I was thinking about my dad, because I was like, "I know my dad. I know he doesn't feel that way." That was another reason why I wanted to interview my dad for the podcast—so we could talk through this. And I remember he said to me, "Look, we lost everything under a Democratic administration, and it didn't get any better for us after that; it only got worse. We tried to get help from the government, we tried to get help from the state, and we either didn't get it or it wasn't enough." Then he said, "After all that, I felt like, for me, in 2016, it was a choice between the devil you know and the devil you don't, and I went with the latter."

Courtney: Wow, that's really profound in itself. Because, like you said, we want to believe the common narrative that all these racist White people are the only reason Trump got elected, which really just takes the blame off the system and puts it back on individuals. That's what liberalism does, right? That was actually a driving force for me in my organizing: I didn't want to vote-shame anyone, I wanted to understand where they were coming from. I'm always critical of these dominant narratives anyway, because I've seen how much powerful people—Democrats and Republicans—lie. So, I'm going to question everything now. I'm not just going to accept whatever explanation the media is giving me for why this or that happened. I'm not going to buy into it just because everybody else is.

That's why I'm so grateful for organizing. It really forced me out of that bubble of thinking that everybody thinks the same way I do, or believes the same thing I do. It forced me to stop thinking that I can know who someone is just based on their politics. I think it's easy for us to kind of paint conservatives as racist, or stupid, or voting against their own interest, instead of just being curious and asking, "Why? What would make a person want to vote for someone like Donald Trump? What are they seeing that I'm not able to see?"

As an organizer, it's been important for me to hold onto that curiosity when I have conversations with people, and to be less judgmental and less sure that my worldview is always the right one.

Max: And that's such a hard skill to learn. In fact, it's one that most people never learn in the first place. That's a real testament to you, to the life path you've taken, and to all the ways that you have turned all your life experience, both the good and the extremely painful, into something that allows you to connect with other human beings on that level. That's a really incredible thing. And hearing you talk made me reflect on the ways my own thinking has shifted over the years. We have pretty similar timelines in that regard. Like you, I came to leftist politics later in life. The recession really was a radicalizing experience for me, and working in factories, warehouses, restaurants, and doing a bunch of other shitty jobs—that really knocked off any lingering ideological dust from my conservative upbringing. But hearing you talk just now kind of helped me realize that when I was a young conservative I hadn't had a whole lot of life experience yet. Then you throw in the fact that I grew up Catholic, which meant that I had a certain understanding about, you know, the cosmic arrangement of things, and the role that mortal sinners like us have in it. That's all to say:

I was basically taught to see the world in a way that assumed that the *system* itself was good and logical, but it was just filled with bad and corrupt people.

Courtney: Mmhmm. Yeah.

Max: And that was also the way I saw other working people. In my mind, the problem was that people weren't good Christians, weren't good citizens, weren't good workers. If they were struggling, it must be because they weren't doing enough on their own to survive in a system that was fundamentally good. However, the older I've gotten, the more experience I've had, the more people I've talked to, the more I've seen what this system does to so many of us, I kind of have the opposite view: I see good people who have been broken by a bad system.

Courtney: God, why are you not an organizer? Are you an organizer? You should totally be! [Laughs.] It's really interesting because I think I grew up with a worldview and an understanding that the system is broken, but I didn't know *how*. I just knew racism—that was the only answer that was provided. It was either racism or you suck as an individual and you just can't cut it. Because if you didn't have racism as a way to explain why you're poor, or why you're experiencing something bad, then the answer is that you, as an individual, just suck, right? Sorry to use such crass terms . . .

Max: Of course! Because that's the only other explanation that you're left with.

Courtney: Exactly. And that's the way we talk about other people in this country. We treat people as "deplorable." Well, I won't say that as a general rule, because it's not like everyone does that, but we definitely do it when it comes to politics. And so, for me, understanding that most people make decisions based on their material conditions and material interests—that doesn't necessarily mean that they're good or bad. It just means they're trying to survive, and some people don't have very many options for survival. Having that understanding has allowed me to have a lot more empathy and compassion for other people, even people who probably wouldn't want me to be alive. You know what I mean? I understand that their hate is probably something *they* don't even fully understand, and if they're provided with a convincing explanation of who the real enemy is, they could change their minds. It's like, "I'm not your enemy. Your gay coworker isn't your enemy. Your boss is." That's another important thing to stress to people, because I don't think people really understand that politics also happens in the workplace. But that's where we all have a lot more in common. That's where they can fight for their rights. That's where their—and our—power is, truly. We don't talk about that at all in the national narrative about who voted for Trump and why.

For me, organizing has helped me be a lot softer in the way that I see the world and in the ways I relate to other human beings in the world—and to myself, honestly.

Max: Man, once again . . . so beautifully put. Let's talk about that a little more. You talked about how you kind of stumbled into the Bernie Sanders movement, then you started working for the Sanders campaign as an organizer. Now that's got me thinking how fucking wild it is that, this time last year, we were still in the middle of the primaries . . . a lot of different possibilities still seemed open at that point. Then, with the dawn of COVID-19, it was like *everything* came crashing down at once, including the progressive hope of a Bernie Sanders presidency. I don't know if any of us will ever fully get over that. For a moment there, it really felt like we had a chance to take the future in a better, less horrifying, war-filled, and planet-killing direction. Could you put yourself back in that position you were in this time last year? As an organizer— but also, you know, as a person, as a parent—what was it like for you going through all of this?

Courtney: Before I talk about me, specifically, I just wanted to bring up something that I've been thinking about a lot lately. American workers don't really get days off, right? We only get like, what, five paid holidays? And that's if you're lucky, if you don't work in the service industry. For me, when the pandemic hit, there was an odd mixture of feelings, because for the first time I felt like I could breathe. Not relax, obviously, because there was a lot of anxiety about not knowing what was going on in the world, and I was just afraid. At the same time, though, I'm not having to go into work every day and sell my body in order to survive. I have to imagine that, for the people who were able to get unemployment, to get that extra $600 a month . . . I think that lifted millions of people out of poverty for a few short months. That must have been the first time a lot of them were able to just stay home and breathe. I think that's what makes this so insidious, too, because it's so confusing how to feel about it.

On the other end of the spectrum, you have people who haven't stayed home and taken precautions and are being shamed for it, which is just another example of individuals being shamed or blamed for big systemic problems that come from the government catastrophically failing us. I guess I wish more people understood that. Think about the situation we're in: They told us to stay home but still go to work, still pay your bills, still struggle. And what we're seeing now is a lot of shaming happening, because the pandemic has been so politicized. So you see a lot of people being shamed for going to hang out with friends, or going out to a bar, traveling, or deciding to live life. Because it didn't really feel like anything stopped for *them*, right? I can understand where they're coming from, because it's like, "Well, why wouldn't they just go on living life? Life didn't stop for them. They still had to go to work and risk getting COVID there, they still had to pay bills, so why would we turn around and take away every reprieve they have to cope with capitalism?" For me, that's been the most insidious part of this whole pandemic. We're making this an individual-focused thing, like we always do. We're shaming people and making them feel guilty, even for just giving someone a hug. And, God, I desperately need a hug, you know? I'm really missing human contact.

Going back to this time last year . . . to paint the full picture, I guess I would also have to explain my day-to-day when I was organizing with Bernie. I was still trying to finish my degree, so I was still going to school and I had my son full-time—and I was dealing with the death of my brother. I think the Bernie campaign gave me that outlet to express my grief in a way that was healthy and that allowed me to just . . . get it out of me and out into the world. Like I said before, it was a way for me to feel like I was creating a world that my brother would have been able to live in, would have wanted to live in. So I did that for six months in Iowa, then we had the February 3 Iowa caucuses, and that was crazy! Actually, a week before the caucuses our entire team had gotten really sick—we all came down with some respiratory virus. They said it was the Influenza B that was going around. But the way that it happened was like: I come into the office one day and an organizer is being sent home because he's not feeling good. I don't think anything of it, I'm just going about my day. Then I take my lunch break at home and I'm like, "Oh, I'm not really feeling good, so I'm gonna lie down and take a nap." I didn't get up for four hours! I was like, "Oh, shit!" [Laughs.] I guess we'll never know, but my theory is that we all got the coronavirus. Because, man, the way that it spread through the office—it was like wildfire. I had never really seen anything like that.

After the Iowa caucuses they redeployed me to Detroit, so I organized in Detroit for about a month until their primary, which was March 10. It was really crazy because I was supposed to go to Chicago after that and organize there, so I was already packing my things and getting ready for that. Then the campaign tells us, "Go home! Drop everything you're doing. Don't go to the hotel we were gonna send you to, just go straight home." That was when we realized, "Oh, shit, it's getting real." I think it was right after the primary here in Michigan that they declared the shutdowns and everything, so it was like . . . it was scary. Because I was still in a place that wasn't my home, I was still staying with my host family, and my primary doctor wasn't there. My son was in Kentucky with his dad, so I had to go to Kentucky, get him, and bring him back with me.

I ended up going back home to Iowa, and we were still organizing with Bernie at that time—all the way until he dropped out in April. And that was probably more devastating than the virus itself. Because at least it still provided something, you know? It was like, "Okay, here's the solution, we just gotta continue to organize and fight." But then he dropped out and Joe Biden was declared the Democratic nominee—I mean, for God's sake, Joe Biden, out of all fucking people! I was like, "Oh, my God! We are fucking going to hell in a handbasket. It's all going to shit, Trump's going to be president again." In my mind I'd completely given up at that point. I was devastated. The only reason I got involved in politics was because of Bernie. So, for me, it felt at the time like there was no other reason to do this work anymore.

This is when it kind of gets interesting, because apparently I just couldn't sit still [laughs], and I decided that I was going to uproot my life from Iowa and move back to Detroit. Because, honestly, I fell in love with

Detroit when I was working here for the campaign. I had met so many great people, and Detroit just has this community feeling to it. It's like . . . capitalism has already destroyed Detroit. The world has already ended in Detroit, so everybody here already knows how hard it is to survive, and they all make sure to work together to survive here. There's just a real sense of camaraderie that I didn't have before, even in Iowa. So I decided I was going to move. I put in my thirty-day notice with my landlord, and I hadn't set up a place to live yet, or a job, or anything like that. I think it was one week before I was set to move that I found a job, and then I found a place the night before I was supposed to move.

Max: Shit, girl! You're cuttin' that real close! [Laughs.]

Courtney: [Laughs.] I was cuttin' it *real* close! I had the U-Haul packed before I even had a place to live. So . . .

Max: I'm over here sweating just thinking about it.

Courtney: Yeah [laughs]. It was exhilarating. Honestly, it gave me something to do and something to look forward to during the pandemic. So I moved my life to Michigan, came here in May. I had my son full-time at the time, and he was doing the virtual school, and that was just such bullshit. When all this first happened and they were trying to figure out virtual schooling, it was a mess. Not that they've figured it out any better now, but it was even worse then. I had just decided, "You know what? We're not doing this." So we just enjoyed our summer, really.

I'll admit, I struggled getting acclimated here. I think it was two months into me living here that the George Floyd riots started. At the time, I was working for an organization that I wasn't particularly psyched about—I was basically organizing for Joe Biden, and I was like, "This fucking sucks." But I needed some sort of income, so I was willing to take anything. Also, I was still going to school, so I was taking online classes and working and being a full-time parent—and still trying to get settled here in Detroit. Those first couple of months were a struggle. It still is. It's been such a roller coaster. But I ended up getting a different job, so now I'm working at a criminal justice organization that works on issues like police brutality and mass incarceration, and that pushes to get people elected who will push our politics on a local level.

I'm much more fulfilled now—and I'm getting paid a lot better than I was before, so that's alleviated a lot of pressure and has helped me cope with the pandemic, because it allows me the flexibility to be able to do what I need to with my son. Now I no longer really have the anxiety that I used to have when it came time to pay bills, because I know that the money's there, and I know that I'm not going to have to work two or three jobs just to make sure we have something to eat. That's really changed the way that I relate to myself—and to the world. Because now I'm also able to, like, do some really necessary mental health work. I've started seeing a nutritionist, which has been life-changing. It's been very eye-opening to realize all the junk that's out there that we're putting into our bodies, and how that affects our emotional states, our mental state, etc. That's another thing I think about now when I think about how the government's impacting us—all these FDA regulations that we don't have on food, all the chemicals they put in food nowadays, and how it really affects you.

So, that's been my personal journey to where I'm at now. But I also wanted to say a little more about the virtual school stuff, because that's been a whole thing on its own . . .

Max: Yeah, let's talk about that. I'm also curious to hear how it's been just being a parent through all of this. I mean, it's a tough time for kids, it's a tough time for parents—it's a lot.

Courtney: It is. It's so hard. God, I don't even know where to start with it. My relationship with my son has completely changed—in good and bad ways. Because now I'm his full-time teacher, and his mom, and I also have to be the sole provider of the house. There's been a lot of relying on TV, or just relying on screens in general, and I hate that. But it's like . . . I don't have very many options right now, because I can't put him in a childcare facility. That would defeat the purpose of staying home. And I don't have very many people I know here who could watch my son for me, so getting breaks is not really a thing for me right now. It's been really stressful. I think that's been the driving force behind my personal journey to just center myself and focus on my mental health. Because, to take this back to politics and my organizing world, I've honestly had to get better at turning some things off and knowing when to say "No." Before this I would do extra organizing voluntarily, until I realized, "Wait, what the fuck am I doing? I'm already working three jobs. I can't do everything!"

Max: I think what you're describing is something that all of us have experienced at some point during this pandemic. At some point or another, we all *knew* how fucked everyone was, because we've seen or experienced ourselves how broken the system was before the pandemic, how little of a safety net there is for people in the "best" of times. When we went into lockdown, I think a lot of us felt that desperate concern for other people, people we knew wouldn't have anywhere to turn, and I think we all felt this drive to respond by doing whatever we could—volunteering, organizing, whatever—because we knew that the government wasn't gonna be there. We knew that "the market" sure as shit wasn't gonna protect people . . . quite the opposite, actually. And so, I understand that impulse to do more work, to organize more, etc. But at the same time, you're already juggling your day job, being a full-time parent, a full-time teacher—you're just doing so much already. I'm glad that you're focusing on caring for yourself. I think we all need to do that. Because at some point during this pandemic we all hit that wall . . .

Courtney: Oh, yeah. I mean, just two weeks ago I was like, "I'm done! I can't do this anymore."

To explain my journey with the virtual schooling stuff: Like I said, at the start of all of this everything was shit. They had no idea what they were doing. And serious kudos to the teachers and the schools for trying to stick through it. But the whole thing is a catastrophic failure because the government really isn't providing any more resources to schools to do this, and schools already don't get the resources they need in general. I'm not saying I have all the solutions or answers to handling this whole thing, but *other* countries are doing more to help their people, right? And it's working! Other countries are paying their citizens $2,000 a month to stay home and they're doing a rent freeze, or a bill freeze so people don't have to worry about how they're going to pay their damn bills in the middle of a pandemic. We did none of that. We barely got any relief. But we still expect people to work, still pay their bills, *and* be the teacher for their kids. It's just so stupid!

Last year, when this was all hitting and everything was chaos, I was like, "Okay, fuck it. I'm not gonna do it. It's society's fault this shit is all fucked up, so I'm not gonna put the pressure on myself to continue this virtual learning nightmare." I decided that we weren't gonna worry about finishing out the rest of last year—and my son was in kindergarten then, so he's young enough to not have to finish the last two months of school. When he started back up this year, Detroit still hadn't figured out what they were going to do with their public schools. They didn't know if they were going to do virtual or in-person schooling. So I decided to keep him enrolled in Kentucky schools, from when he was staying with his dad. At that point I was going back and forth co-parenting with his dad. I would drive to meet him halfway—in total, it was a six-hour drive—and we'd rotate every three weeks. Here's the setup that we had: The school would do online instruction for an hour a day—from like 9:30 to 10:30—and then they would post assignments that we would do together. They had other classes that he needed to go to, but I'd decided that I was just going to do reading and math with him—we were going to do our assignments for those and that was it. And so, I would finish doing his school stuff with him at noon, then I'd be able to do my work. It took us a while to get into a good routine with that.

So, I did have somewhat of a break and some help from his dad, until I found out that he wasn't doing the schoolwork with our son because he works two jobs outside of the home. He was struggling to keep up with it. We had a conversation about it and we decided he was going to stay with me, since I work at home full-time and I'm able to actually sit and do the schoolwork with him. The plan was to enroll him in Detroit Public Schools—that way, when they go back to in-person learning, he'd already be enrolled and all that good stuff. So, I enrolled him and, you know, they . . . I struggle with it, because I want to be delicate in my assessment. I *know* that the teachers are really trying—his teacher at the Detroit school was so helpful and would text or call to make sure that we got set up and everything—but the School Board policy for the districts was that the kids needed to be online from 8:30 a.m. to 3:40 p.m. They had to have their cameras on and they needed to be tested damn near every day, it seemed like. It was a lot . . . it was a lot. We did that for a good month, and we literally cried every single day afterward. I mean, every day, by one o'clock, my son's asking me, "Are we done yet? Can I be done? Can I just . . ." And he's seven! He can't read or write on his own yet, so I would have to sit with him literally the entire day and basically be in school with him and help him do his work. Because that's the only way that the teacher can tell whether or not they're doing their work and give them a grade—by having them write it out. But you're dealing with first graders! They can't really write yet. So, I'm trying to teach him how to do all of this and help him through it, and I can tell it was causing him so much anxiety. And our relationship was just becoming so torn because I had to be his teacher now. I had to be the one to make him pay attention, to have him sit down and do all of these things—and to crack the whip, I guess? I would get really frustrated, *he* would get really frustrated, and it was just . . . it was a disaster. God bless the teachers right now. They deserve to be paid so much better than what they are getting. I'm appalled that we're putting them through this and not paying them enough.

After we would get done with his school day at 3:40 I would then have to start *my* workday. Basically, I would be online until ten, eleven o'clock at night—some nights I would fall asleep at my computer. It got to a point where I was like, "I don't even want to go to bed," because I knew I would have to wake up and do it all over again. On top of all that, of course, I'm still dealing with the other stresses of living in capitalism, like arguing with shitty landlords who aren't coming to do repairs. Every time I'm dealing with shit like that and it feels like every little thing is going wrong, I'm like, "Fuck, I don't have time for this! I don't even have the space to breathe right now! How am I supposed to do this?" So, just a week ago, I decided that I was going to pull my son out of school and just homeschool him instead, which was a really tough decision, because I know that public school funding is dependent on how many kids are enrolled. But as much as I want to support public funding for his school, I also know that my material conditions right now do not allow that. I guess this comes back to why understanding the material conditions people live under, understanding how and why people make the decisions they do, is so important. It really helps to soften the guilt that I was feeling over pulling him out of public school. Ever since I did that, though, there's just been such a huge weight lifted off my shoulders. Now I'm working on reconnecting with my son again and just kind of . . . healing. The whole thing was a really traumatic experience, to be honest. I don't know if I did it justice by my explanation, but it was a fucking nightmare.

Max: Oh, I wouldn't worry about that. From this end it sounded like a fucking nightmare . . .

Courtney: Ok! [Laughs.] I'm just making sure that I'm painting a real clear picture here, because I need people to know this shit is not okay—what we're putting parents through, what we're putting teachers through, and what we're putting our children through. I'm so angry at our government for the way that it's failed us, and I'm angry that we elected Joe Biden, who's not going to fucking do anything! Hopefully he'll prove me wrong . . . maybe . . . I don't know. He could be the next Lyndon B. Johnson. Who knows? I doubt it.

6. Kyle Killebrew

I'm Kyle Norman Killebrew. I'm thirty-three years old. I'm a union sheet metal worker out of Louisville, Kentucky, Local 110 [International Association of Sheet Metal, Air, Rail and Transportation Workers]. That's pretty much the gist. I've lived in Louisville my whole entire life. And I've been doing union sheet metal work for coming up on sixteen years now, since I graduated from high school. Started three weeks right out of high school . . .

Max: Damn, *three weeks* out of high school?

Kyle: [Laughs.] Yeah.

Max: Man, you didn't even give yourself a chance to get wild after high school, eh?

Kyle: I was able to get a little wild. I had a bunch of friends in fraternities and shit. I was just the one who always had a little bit of money in my pocket—they were all broke college kids.

Max: [Laughs.]

Kyle: And I was always working Saturday nights—lotta Friday nights too. I worked a lot of Saturdays in the beginning but, hell, we hardly never work Sundays because that's all double time. But yeah, it was fun. I don't regret it at all. Like I said, I had a lot of friends in fraternities and they did the college thing for three or four years. Now they're all union pipefitters, union plumbers, HVAC service techs, etc. They did the college thing and they was like, "Ehhh, I partied my ass off. I'm gonna go do skilled trades now." [Laughs.]

Max: [Laughs.] Shockingly, as we all find out sooner or later, partying doesn't pay the bills.

Kyle: Well, some people get lucky enough to get a job like that. But the rest of us . . . we gotta do some form of actual work.

Max: Right, right. And you said you're born and raised in Louisville, yeah? You got deep family roots there?

Kyle: Yeah. I got family in other places too—got some family in Missouri. If you stretch from around Kansas City to Louisville, we got family all in-between. I'm a Chiefs fan and we got the Super Bowl coming up here, so: Go Chiefs! [Laughs.] But yeah, we're pretty thick here in the north-central part of Kentucky—you know, Louisville and the surrounding areas.

Max: Were you raised in a union household? Or are you the first sheet metal worker in the family? Obviously, when it comes to big industries in Kentucky, a lot of people know about the coal mining. But Louisville itself is a major city with a number of different industries with union workforces.

Kyle: I'm actually a second-generation sheet metal worker. My mom, believe it or not—she's retired from the Sheet Metal Workers union. She did twenty-three years. She had to go out early, but she was a union sheet metal worker, a journeyman. And her dad, my grandfather—he was UAW [United Auto Workers]. We got two Ford plants in Louisville: one where they make Super Duties and one where they make the Escapes. He worked at both of 'em. He did forty-some odd years . . . forty-two or forty-three years total at those two plants.

So, yeah, we're pretty thick in with the unions here and just collective bargaining in general. I mean, I got some family members who sit on the other side of the negotiating table, but even they're still for unions. You know what I'm sayin'? It just . . . it just means a lot. It's hard to explain it to people, but it's just totally different, man, the way it's approached here.

Your average worker feels like they're just another number and this and that. With a union, though, if someone tries to tell you you're just another number, you're like, "Well, hold your horses there, Hoss."

Max: [Laughs.] Hell yeah. "Well, we're a little more than that!"

Kyle: And we got the contract to show it! So, yeah, we're a pretty thick union family—pretty thick Democratic family too, to be honest with you. We got a lot of family members who are Republicans, don't get me wrong. But being union—it's definitely laid the roots of our political views as well.

Max: Let's talk about that a little bit. I'm super interested in this, even just from a personal standpoint, because I grew up in a pretty conservative, Catholic, non-union household. And it was only later in life that I realized that there was a pretty even split in our family. One side of the family, the Mexican side, was pretty heavily Democrat, and almost everyone on that side of the family had union jobs. On the other side of the family, though, mainly the White side—they were all Republicans and had non-union jobs. We were the mixed-race family in the middle, but we grew up on the conservative, non-union side. I didn't come to the movement until much later in life. For a long time I was very steeped in that anti-union culture, you know? I heard all the bullshit about teachers' unions, "lazy teachers," "impossible-to-fire teachers," yadda, yadda, yadda.

Kyle: Sure.

Max: That shit was just a mainstay of L.A. talk radio and the world I grew up in. But I'm curious to hear more about what that looked like for you growing up, even in your own family. Was union politics something that was discussed a lot at the table or at family gatherings? Was being union and leaning more Democrat the norm when you were going to school and talking to your friends and their families?

Kyle: Oh, yeah. But just to touch back really quick on what you said before about growing up Catholic . . . I was raised Catholic. K–12, I went to l'il private, Catholic schools. That was a big thing for my mom and dad, for me and my sister to go to the best Catholic schools. Like I said, my mom was union. My dad wasn't, but he was definitely pro-union. It really was the norm for us. From the time I was little—it was so weird—I always felt like me and my friends were older souls, because I was so interested in politics when I was younger, watching the late-night shows like Bill Maher, even Dennis Miller when he used to be on HBO. I always kind of wanted to hear what one side's take was, then hear the other's. But when it came to being union and being in a union household, I never understood why people were *anti-union*. If you're not in a union, whatever, it's fine. Everybody's got to work. I was never brought up to be like, "Oh, the non-union guys—those are rats," or, "those are scabs." It was like, "No, those are working people too. We want them to come join our group, because they can live better and it'll be better on them in the long run."

The side of Louisville we live on—it's the working-class side, the southwest side. And there were a lot of kids I grew up with who went to the Catholic schools. A lot of the families whose kids attended those schools—they worked in one of the two Ford plants, or they worked at what used to be Philip Morris, which left in the early 2000s. Or they worked in a building trade, or one of the parents was a nurse, or something like that. I know that's not always the case at other Catholic schools, private schools, and other places. But what I'm saying is: Nobody was really well-to-do. And we was always just like, "Hey, work union, live better." It's kind of like the Walmart slogan, "Save money, live better." But it was more like, "Hey, you work union, this is what you got: You got your pension, you got your health insurance, you got unemployment." And there was a whole other list of perks too. I never understood the whole anti-union sentiment, this whole attitude like, "Oh, unions want these higher wages, but if everybody was union then it'd drive inflation up" and this and that. When I hear people saying all this I'm just like, "What?" [Laughs.] Like, "Someone explain this." I mean, hell, Jeff Bezos, he's doing well—I'm sure he could pay his people a little bit more. It blows my mind the amount of wealth that's out there, and the amount of struggling that goes on with this modern human condition we have here.

Max: Right.

Kyle: It's mind-blowing. It really is.

Max: Yeah, it's so transparently obscene and perverse that we almost have to spend extra time and effort convincing ourselves that it's not. Like, we can't stare the monster in the face, because it's too ridiculous and too horrifying to confront head on.

I think that, for my part, my experience with that anti-union sentiment was more cultural than anything. Like I said, there was a lot of anti-union culture that I grew up with—and with a lot of that stuff, the older I got, the more I realized, "Oh, this is just straight propaganda from the ruling class. This doesn't benefit anybody but them."

Kyle: Sure.

Max: But I will say that growing up as a mixed-race kid in Southern California, there was some profound and complex stuff there that conservatism, as it was presented to me, really tapped into. Take my dad, for instance, Jesus. He's a Mexican immigrant—grew up dirt poor in Tijuana before being separated from most of his family and moved in with a foster family in California. He became a citizen in the early 1980s, and he voted for Reagan. My mom was always kind of a Reagan Democrat, now she's more Independent. But, looking back, I can see how and why my dad was so sold on the American dream. I mean, he lived it! For a time. We ended up losing everything in the recession, like a lot of families did, and I think that his politics have changed since then. But the point is: He very much had, and my parents very much raised us with, this sense that we would all have to make our own path in life. And the things that were going to really matter were talking well, learning a lot, and working hard.

Kyle: Right.

Max: As a more conservative family, there was almost an unspoken understanding we were raised with—especially when it came to the question of race—that the world itself is unfair, but you can't control that. You just have to focus on what you *can* control, and that's where the emphasis on hard work and self-determination came in. I think that's probably what kept me as a conservative throughout high school and into my early twenties—this notion that people are gonna judge me, the world itself is gonna be unfair, but if I put my nose down, work hard, and just focus on myself, I could get ahead in life. It's easier, and often a lot less painful, to wrap your head around *that* than to try to understand why the world is so cruel and unjust and why hardly anyone does anything to change it. I'm not a conservative anymore, obviously, but I think that's why my former self was so drawn to it. The focus on personal responsibility, hard work, and getting ahead—it's appealing. It makes you feel more empowered to shape your own destiny, and who doesn't want to feel that? But the older you get, the more you realize how rigged the fucking system is and how hard and deliberately impossible it is for most of us to succeed individually playing such a rigged game.

Kyle: Yeah, I agree. And I would say, too, if you watch old footage of Ronald Reagan or even George H.W. Bush, and you listen to the way they talk—it's hard to really disagree with what they're saying, with the kind of tone they use and everything else. You listen to them and you're like, "Yeah! Let's work hard. Let's do this." And the thing is: I don't think anybody is saying, "Oh, I want a bunch of shit for free," or that we're just holding hands out like, "Gimme, gimme, gimme." Growing up, I never felt like politicians needed to do anything *for* me or my mom, my dad, or our family. We didn't need anything from them—we just needed politicians to *not* do bad stuff.

Max: [Laughs.]

Kyle: That was the biggest thing. Just like with "right to work" laws or, as we always say, "right to work for less" laws. My mom was always so excited that Kentucky wasn't one of those "right to work" states like Tennessee, Alabama, Georgia, Texas, and all these states to the south of us. And Kentucky was where the strength started. From there you had Indiana, Ohio, West Virginia, and all these places that fought to keep those laws away. We just didn't want them to come here and break down the unions with this "right to work for less" shit, which basically ensures that there's no money (through union dues) to do collective bargaining. Because you need that money to be effective—you have to have union officers and officials, and sometimes, when contract negotiations get tough, you got to call in your lawyers. And lawyers aren't cheap, especially the good ones. I knew that years and years ago in high school. If I ever did get into a debate with someone who was from a more conservative household, it was always like, "Well, *my* family's not union and they do just fine." Look, that's great, but there might come a time at your job when they say, "We can't afford to give a raise this year. We can't afford this or that." And if that happens, what're you gonna do? You gonna rally everybody there and walk out? No, you're just gonna take it.

When things are good you can be union, non-union, sure, whatever. When shit hits the fan, though? Then it's like, "Whoa, whoa, whoa, hold on a minute." I don't know. Like I said, I always agreed with that "Yeah, let's work hard!" attitude, but . . . just don't come after me. Don't come here and try to make it harder for me to live. Don't make it to where my work is meaningless and devalued all because you signed this law that says, "Hey, nobody has to pay union dues. Isn't that great?" It's just . . . it's frustrating.

Speaking of that, I remember January 5, 2017. Kentucky, for the first time in ninety-five years, had a Republican House of Representatives. And I was there in the House chambers that night, in the rotunda with a bunch of other people from labor, watching all these representatives giving their speeches. They was getting rid of prevailing wage, putting the "right to work" law in, and saying things like, "You don't have to pay union dues no more!" You had this fresh House of brand new, been-on-the-job-for-four-or-five-days representatives all telling their stories about why Kentucky needed these laws and saying things like, "I have an uncle who's a union millwright!" and "My brother has been a union operator for thirty years!" And I'm sitting there thinking, "Then why would you vote to pass this thing through? What the hell are you doing?" It blew my mind. I was like, "Oh, my God! You're just spitting in all our faces."

The thing about these laws is: It don't affect you right away, but ten, fifteen years down the road you're gonna feel it. That's what it's designed to do. That's what really worries me. That's why these last four or five years I've gotten so into politics. I always would do phone banks and this and that come election time, and I've walked for certain candidates I felt strongly about—people I've had good conversations with. But at this point it's like, man, if you live in this country, or anywhere in the world, you can't afford to not get involved anymore. You gotta get up off the bench.

Max: I feel that, man, and I think you're exactly right. God, all the "right to work" stuff is just infuriating. It's the biggest fucking swindle in history.

Kyle: [Laughs.] Oh, yeah.

Max: First of all, the name itself is just the most misleading piece-of-shit slogan ever. And just like you said, this is exactly what "right to work" does. It sells workers on this short-term thing that is presented as a gain for them. They're like, "Oh, we're keeping Big Bad Labor from taking money out of your paycheck for union dues. We're the ones who are really looking out for you!" Especially for people who have never had a union job and are barely scraping by on their wages as it is, that's a very effective scare tactic. But they don't ever tell you what union dues are for or how they help you and your coworkers. They just paint it as money that's disappearing from your paycheck. And like you said, that short-term "gain" may seem nice, but then you end up in those situations where, if you have a down year, or if management starts making decisions that you have no say over, you start realizing just how unprotected you are and how *alone* you are in the workplace. By then it's too late—they've already won. They've already taken the safety net away, and it's just a freefall for all of us.

Kyle: Yeah.

Max: I'll tell you something, man. That's one thing that has become very clear in the conversations I've been having with people for this book and for the podcast I do. Especially during the COVID-19 pandemic, when I'm talking to union and non-union workers about this stuff, it's very clear which side generally feels more protected and which side generally feels like they're completely on their own.

Kyle: Oh, yeah. And that "right to work" slogan, man . . . when it comes to wording, Republicans are just the best. Are you "pro-life?" Are you against the "death tax?" You know what I'm sayin'? They can really make it to where anything sounds unattractive, no matter what it is, no matter what signals they're trying to send. They'll word it perfectly and just keep a straight face and hit you with it. And some people eat it up. But I will say this: I've seen a big shift in the last ten years with circles I run around in, even people I grew up with who were more conservative. Views are definitely changing, especially if you spend any time out in the real world. You got mortgages, or you have to pay off some kind of predatory loan, or you just find yourself in a bind and you need this or that—you gotta deal with all this stuff and you run into things where you're like, "How the hell is this even legal?" That's when you really start to see that politics is a big deal.

Max: I think what you described about "right to work" being this big fucking con that we don't feel the full weight of until years down the road—that same principle seems to be at play in the economy writ large.

Kyle: Right.

Max: But I think people are catching on to that. You mentioned that, even in the circles you run in, you've noticed a shift in folks' attitudes over the past ten years or so. I've noticed the same thing. I mean, when we were growing up, I never could have imagined that a candidate like Bernie Sanders would be as popular as he is now, let alone that so many people would openly and proudly call themselves socialists. I've been wondering why that is and where that mood shift is coming from. Why are so many people—and not just Millennials and Zoomers—from so many parts of the country responding to this? And on top of all that, you've got this growing popular support for the labor movement. Labor unions are more popular now than they've been in over half a century! There's definitely something going on here. Maybe people are waking up.

I think a lot of it comes down to that same thing you described about living in a "right to work" state—when you've had so many of your protections and rights as a worker stripped away but you don't even know it yet. They take those things away from us during the "boom" years so we don't even notice, but you really feel their absence when the "bust" comes. If you take that same principle and apply it to society as a whole . . . that's kind of the world that you and I grew up in. The economy was doing pretty well in the '90s and early 2000s, then everything just fucking went to shit with the recession and working people were the ones left holding the bag. It's almost like the ruling class couldn't help itself after that. They just kept taking and taking, and they made sure the "recovery" since 2008 has basically only benefited them while things have either stayed the same or gotten worse for so many of us. If they were smart, if they didn't want to spawn a whole bunch of socialists and labor enthusiasts, they would have at least tried to keep that dream of social mobility alive, but they couldn't help themselves. Now, when so many people are left with so few options to get by, let alone reach a comfortable middle-class existence, that's radicalizing people a little bit. That's why you've got more people saying, "Maybe socialism isn't so bad," and, "Maybe we do need unions." It's like we're all looking around and we're realizing how little recourse we have, especially if we don't have a union or if we live in an anti-worker state. We're only now realizing just how far behind we've been playing and how stacked the deck is against us.

Kyle: Oh, yeah. I think that's a big reason why Trump lost in 2020 too. It's the same reason Carter didn't get reelected. Reagan asked people, "Are you better off than you were four years ago?" and people said, "Well, fuck no. I'm not." With Trump, people asked the same question: "Am I better off than I was four years ago?" I think a lot of people who voted for him last time either sat out or they voted for Biden this time around, because they were like, "No, I'm not better. This shit is not better."

Max: Right.

Kyle: On a personal level, our local here in Kentucky, Local 110, has gotten so much stronger since I've been in. And I'm talking about everything, from little things like the attendance at the union meetings, to the things we do outside of work like going out and putting ourselves out there in the community, doing things for the community. We've got to, like, sell ourselves to people who aren't just family members or dues-paying members. We've gotta be out there like, "Hey, look, this is what we're doing." We're putting on these fishing derbies, we do the Paducah Labor Day Parade, which is the largest ongoing Labor Day parade this side of the Mississippi—it's been going on for frickin' 140 years or something. Well, it might not be that long. It might be 127 years. I don't know. But we're selling ourselves, you know? We're here, we're there, we're at the State Fair—we got our booth where we're giving shit away that we made, like these nice tool trays. We're just really trying to be like, "Hey, we're a union, we're not bad. Here's a fishing pole and a tackle box for your kid. Have fun today. Hopefully y'all catch some fish." Just little shit like that. But I think it does go a long way in the grand scheme of it all.

Max: Oh yeah, I bet it does! If I would have had that kind of presence in my childhood, I think I would have thought a lot differently about unions.

Kyle: Yeah.

Max: Speaking of the union, let's go back to when you first got this job. You were just saying that, over the years that you've been there in Local 110 and doing this kind of work, you've seen the changes firsthand and you've experienced them yourself. Take us back to the beginning and let's talk about what those changes looked like through your own eyes. We already talked about how you got this job three weeks out of high school, while a number of your friends were going off to college. So, was college not a big thing for you? With your mom being a sheet metal worker, did you know that this was what you wanted to do?

Kyle: Initially, I was gonna go to Louisville Technical Institute. I done paid my 10 percent down, 50 percent down, whatever it was. I was gonna go be a marine mechanic. I wanted to work on boats and jet skis. My family got a little place down at a lake like an hour and a half outside of Louisville, southwest of Louisville. I always liked going down there, and I remember thinking, "You know what? That would be a cool job, working on boats all through the spring and summer—hell, even in the winter months. People could bring their boat to me and I'll fix it up." That was my initial plan. I made the down payment on the technical program and I was just planning to work down there by the lake for the summer, make a little extra money. I was gonna try to do it sporadically here and there in between school, and that school actually wasn't too far away from where I worked. My class was supposed to start around the first part of October, I think, but they sent me a letter around the first part of September and they sent my check back. The letter was like, "We only had four people sign up for this, so we're discontinuing the Louisville program. With dropping enrollment year after year, we can't afford to keep it open." And it was only, like, a two-year program—eighteen months, maybe. And so, I was like, "Shit." I had the option: I could go down to Chattanooga or go down to Daytona and do the same program. But I was like, "Nah, I don't really want to do that. I'll just stay here and figure it out."

Then, like a couple weeks before I turned eighteen, I was at the job I'm at now—I was just a cleanup boy in the beginning, what they called a "pre-apprentice." You gotta work your way up to doing sheet metal work. I was like, "I'm gonna do this. If I get in and start now, by the time I'm twenty-three I'll be a journeyman." And I did it. I took my test at the end of October, turned in all my paperwork, did my interview, and then I waited. Eventually I got moved up from pre-apprentice and became an apprentice. It took me a long time, though. I was number four on the waiting list, but the economy was slowing down. This was at the end of 2005, and you could really start to see the foreboding that was coming on with the recession. But I got taken on eleven months after I'd signed up, so I had just turned nineteen by the time I was going into the apprentice program. My first two weeks working there were, like, the worst two weeks of my life. I hated it . . .

Max: [Laughs.]

Kyle: But when I got that first paycheck on Friday . . . I mean, I'd always had a job, but I went from making $4.75 an hour working on this farm in our neighborhood, cutting mint for the Kentucky Derby (we also did different greens and turnips and stuff), to having a job making $10 an hour. Plus working overtime—coming in on Saturdays, making time-and-a-half all day. When you're seventeen or eighteen that's a big deal. Then they ended up giving me a $2.50 pay raise after being there for like four weeks!

They were like, "Man, you're really killing it, you're working hard. We're gonna give you some more money." So I was like, "Well, shit, this ain't bad."

Like I said, I didn't know that this is what I was gonna do. I was never like, "Ah, I want to go to college and be an engineer or a doctor," you know? I always liked working with my hands. That's why I thought, "Hey, I like working on my truck and tinkering with motors and stuff. That might be a good career." But I didn't want to be an auto mechanic. I wanted to work on something that was specialized because you can do alright working that way. You got a niche, you get in the right place, you could make really good money. Eventually, sheet metal was my trade of choice. It was what my mom did, and now I got four different cousins who are sheet metal workers. I got one cousin who is still an apprentice, but the rest of them are all journeymen. And my brother-in-law—he's a journeyman sheet metal worker too. It's become quite the family affair. We all work at different companies and we're all spread out through the local. Local 110 represents workers at a number of different shops in the area. It's really cool.

Max: That's so cool, man. I was laughing to myself when you were saying that, as a high schooler, if you're making a little over minimum wage you feel like you're rolling in it. That's so true. You don't have a whole lot of expenses, so it's just cash in your pocket, right? But then, when you get paid at this apprenticeship—even though, like you were saying, the first two weeks were the worst of your life—you see your paycheck and you're like, "Oh, shit!" [Laughs.] How big was that first paycheck? Was it way more than you expected?

Kyle: Oh, yeah. In 2005 my first few paychecks were for like $299. That's the pay rate I was getting: $299 a week, *plus* I was paying into and had my own health insurance. And I was paying into this pension thing that I was going to have access to when I was fifty-five, if I stuck with the job. But, you know, no eighteen-year-old thinks about that shit.

Max: [Laughs.] Right.

Kyle: And then, like I said, once I was in the apprentice program I got another raise and I was like, "Okay!" As a pre-apprentice, they really didn't let me do a whole lot until I turned eighteen, because it was a liability thing. But once I turned eighteen I got to start using power tools and doing all that other stuff, working for this journeyman, working for that journeyman, or learning from a couple apprentices and just letting them tell me what to do, because these are guys who've been in it for a few years. Then, next thing you know, I was an apprentice myself. I was the youngest apprentice down there, I think, for two and a half years. Then two guys came along who were a year younger than me. But yeah, I full-on got on board with it and I was just always trying to make it better—the work, the union, all of it.

Max: That's awesome, man. And speaking of the work, one of the things I always love asking about is what goes into the job itself. Because I have no fucking idea what it's like to be a sheet metal worker. I'm not a journeyman. And I imagine a lot of folks who are going to be reading this will probably have no clue what that's like either. So, from those first two horrible weeks as a pre-apprentice to moving your way up the ranks all the way to where you are now, what's the work been like? What's a regular week on the job look like for you?

Kyle: I guess the first thing to point out is that I've taken on other positions throughout the union as well. Like, ones that I can do while still keeping my main job. I guess you could say I'm one of their lead journeymen. They might put me on a project with other . . . actually, let me back up so I can give you a little background.

The company I work for is called Vendome Copper & Brass Works and we are the largest distillation manufacturer in the United States. We're coppersmiths. Yeah, we're union sheet metal workers, but we specialize in copper and brass and different alloys that your typical guy who's got a welding rig isn't going to be able to tackle. So, our company has to invest a lot in every single one of their employees to get them to the point where they can trust you to handle a pallet of seven sheets of copper—sheets that cost $8,000 a piece. It's outrageous. It's all gotta come from Germany, but anyway . . . We build whatever, whether it's a moonshine system, a big beer still system, or a big column system for a big player like a Jack Daniels or a Jim Beam . . .

Max: You're talking about, like, those big fucking distillery-type drums?

Kyle: Yes.

Max: Nice.

Kyle: And we build all the equipment for them. We don't mess a whole lot with the dry grain side of the process. The stuff we make is for when it hits the cooking side . . . so, the pressure vessels. We make a lot of stainless-steel vessels, whether it be fermenters, beer wells, mash cookers, yeast cookers, or anything like that, all the way down to the condensers, the spirit safes, and all the real fancy ornamental things.

If you get some time, look us up. It really is a family-owned company. They're in their fourth generation right now, their doors have been open since, like, 1903. They got a really good niche going on. And we're smack dab in the center of the bourbon boom too. That seemed to slow down for a little bit last year, obviously, because of COVID, but they've really invested a lot in the company and it's just been growing year after year. I've seen it—there'd be times when you'd think we were about to get slow and then *boom*, another major project would come up and we would be slammed for seven months again. Then we would go back down to forty hours a week for two or three months, then next thing you know it's fifty-eight hours a week, or the boss is saying, "You guys gotta work seven twelves for the next six weeks so we can finish this project—they gotta hit these deadlines."

Now, having the kind of tenure I got there, they might put me on a project like the one I'm working on now, which we're shipping tomorrow. It's four fermenters and it's for a distillery down in Gatlinburg, Tennessee, called Sugarlands. There were five other guys working with me and everybody had their roles, and when everybody would get their parts done we put the fermenters together. And when it comes to fermenters, there's not really much to them, but there is. There's a lot on the engineering side, and there's a lot when it comes to the small, fine details. The reason why our customers come back to us again and again is the little things we do differently that other manufacturers won't do. We kinda got our own signature, I guess you'd say, on all our equipment. And a lot of families have done really well for themselves because of this product we make. And when you strip it all down, it's cuz this is a union product. Yeah, they put a lot in n the engineering side too, but we hold ourselves to the highest account-ability and we make sure that everything is perfect, *boom*, dead nuts, to a tee, when it goes out the door. And when the customer sends an email, it's always gonna be a good email, like, "Hey! All this equipment's great; it looks beautiful in here. We're getting our fifteen gallons a second of proof alcohol," or whatever—just depends on what size the distillery is. We do a lot of work at Anheuser-Busch as well, and they're *the* player when it comes to beer in the United States.

Max: Yeah! And you're right. It's wild to think about—and I guess I hadn't thought about this until right now when you mentioned it—but bourbon was hot as shit up until the pandemic hit. I remember seeing so many peo-ple making new bourbons, so many people buying bourbon—hell, *I* was buying new bourbons. I love bourbon. The bourbon craze was very real. It just feels like such a long time ago now. But it was only like a year ago . . .

Kyle: [Laughs.] Yeah, like eleven months ago . . .

Max: Eleven months ago, right. And going beyond just bourbon distill-eries, I'm thinking about all these different types of distilleries out there: small ones, big ones, from the boutique microbreweries all the way up to Anheuser-Busch. When you think about how those places operate, you think about all those things you were talking about—the barrels that they store whiskey in, those huge copper drums, and all the fancy machinery that ferments the shit, distills the shit, bottles the shit, etc. That's what's so cool about this, right? We think about those distilleries, and that machin-ery, as the place where the good stuff is made—whiskey, beer, whatever. But we rarely ever think, "Well, where is *that* stuff made? Who makes the equipment that makes the stuff we consume? Where does *that* come from?" And it's you! *You're* the ones who are making it.

Kyle: Yeah! And you know what's crazy? Before the pandemic, two or three times a week there'd be a tour come through our shop with people who are bourbon connoisseurs, or people who are interested in opening up a mom-and-pop distillery in, say, Bethesda, Maryland, or someplace like that. Just all kinds of people from all over the country—all over the world, really—will come through. We've even had some pretty big-name celebrities who were involved in this or that distillery or making this special brew. They usually don't bring them in during the week, but if they were in town they'd come down on a Saturday while half the shop was working and they'd get to walk around the facility. And all those Discovery Channel show people come through, like the one guy with the long dreadlocks, one of those moonshiners who's got the bar up there in Sturgis—I forget his name. It's pretty cool. And there are a lot more people now who're like, "Oh, where's all this handmade copper equipment coming from? Who is behind it? Where does that stuff come from?" It's coming from Germany, Ireland, Scotland, and the United States—and when it comes from the United States it's probably coming from us.

Max: That's so cool, man. And clearly there are a lot of different skills and tasks that go into that, right? I guess it depends on the project you're working on, but even from what you were describing it's obvious that there's a good amount of welding, a good amount of assembly, etc. Could you talk a little bit about all the different types of tasks and tools and stuff that goes into that work?

Kyle: To anybody looking from the outside it's gonna look like an assembly line. You got three or four guys that are working with these four pieces of equipment—like a shear, for example. All your metals are coming in off trucks and they get labeled. When prints get handed out a guy over in the warehouse will bring pallets of metal up. You'll have your print and you'll shear it all down. You put it through the shear, you stomp out the sizes you need for this and that, something needs to be welded here or there . . . a whole lot goes into it. It's a lot of welding, but it's more than just the welding. You might be laying out something around the tank and putting a skin over it. You might have an insulation jacket or something in there, and you're gonna lay out another piece of metal, and you're gonna drill a hole in it, etc. Your math better be on, too, and you're going to want to have it checked, then checked again by quality control, and *then* you can go ahead and do it. We also do brazing, and we use some other methods too.

But yeah, it's a whole lot of welding and grinding and going up and down ladders, and everything gets polished to a tee so there's no scratches in the metal or anything like that. Other manufacturers—they don't care about the little details and stuff. They'll just be like, "Aw, hell, in six months' time, after it's been running, this part of the machine's gonna change colors" or whatever. But, you know, the little things we do—I think that's what really separates us in the long haul.

Max: Damn, that is really fucking cool. Do you know what I was doing while I was listening to you describe all that? I was side-eyeing the bookshelf that I built myself, which, up until this moment, I was very proud of [laughs].

Kyle: [Laughs.]

Max: It's such an imprecise, backyard-project kind of bookshelf—it's a total hodgepodge of different types of wood. I remember there was an old house being renovated up the road, so one day I just went rummaging through the torn-out panels and frames and collected enough shit to build a bookshelf. But damn, thinking about just how precise you guys have to be when you're doing this work, how in sync you have to be, how you have to adjust to all the specifications that clients are giving you . . . it's very daunting. And I guess that's why, like you said, you need that union standard.

Kyle: I will say this: Wood is not my craft. In my opinion, wood is a lot harder than metal, because if you're a little bit off with welding you can fill it in and blend it all in and make it look like you didn't mess up nothing. With wood you can't do that. But that's the way you learn, though! You just gotta get out there and you gotta build it. And that's good. I bet you that bookcase is fine. It's doing its job.

Max: It's doing its job [laughs]. I can say that much. It's got books on it and it hasn't fallen apart, so I'm happy.

Kyle: Right. There ya go.

Max: Well, we've kind of already started to eke into the timeline of events that brought us into this strange new reality of the COVID-19 era. Could we try to go back to that time when things started changing, both on the business side of things at Vendome Copper & Brass Works and on the more personal side with you, your wife, your family, etc.? Can you put yourself back in that time period when you started to realize, "Oh, shit, this is happening . . . and it's here."

Kyle: Two weeks before Christmas 2019, I come home from work and turn on CNN. I'm sitting there watching them talk about an outbreak of this unidentified, flu-like thing in Wuhan, China. And somebody—I wanna say it was Jake Tapper—was talking about it and asking this guest, "What are they going to do?" And the guest says, "They're talking about maybe doing a lockdown." So then Jake's like, "Whoa, a lockdown! What do you mean, a lockdown?" And whoever he was talking to was like, "Well, lock down the entire city of Wuhan." And, you know, Wuhan's got a population the size of New York City. And ol' Jake's like, "That's crazy! But hopefully everything works out good for them." That was right around the time leading up to Christmas. I remember seeing that and thinking, "That's eleven million people! You're not gonna be able to lock down eleven million people! You're not gonna be able to tell eleven million people they can't leave their house."

That's about the time I started watching it more closely. I remember turning off the TV and going to work on my truck up at my uncle's garage and we were talking about it, because he'd been hearing about it too. I think even Sean Hannity—my uncle's a big Sean Hannity and Rush Limbaugh guy—was talking about it that day. I remember my uncle saying, "Oh, yeah, that city over there in China—they're gonna lock that thing down for months till they can get this under control. People are dying right and left." And then my other uncle was like, "Yeah, that shit would never work over here." But I said, "Well, if it's killing people like that they'd have to try something, especially if it made its way here." And that was kind of the end of it. We went on to another topic.

Then, sure enough, two-and-a-half or three months later, I wouldn't even go up there to my uncle's garage. I was just going to work and coming home, trying to pinpoint the best times to go to the grocery store and all that. Come early March it was clear that this shit was really going down. But, man, when all that started happening it was really odd because, given the industry we're in and the work we do, it was half and half talking to guys at work. Certain guys were saying, "We're not 'essential' workers. Governor Beshear is saying we need to stay home and this and that. To hell with coming to work—I'm not gonna get this shit." And I know it's serious. I mean, it's always been serious. I've known a lot of people who've succumbed to this, people who lost their lives. More people than from any other thing I can think of, at least in that short amount of time. I remember I had to talk to my wife about it. I told her, "Well, this guy and this guy— they're just gonna file for unemployment." And our company . . . we was talking to the owners, we was saying, "Hey, what do y'all got going on? Are y'all gonna lay us off? What are you gonna do?" And they said, "Oh, we're just gonna play it by ear day-to-day, see what the governor says and change our policies if we need to." And they did.

We was getting a new three- or four-page packet every few days for about a month there. We had approximately sixty-five union members at work at the start of the pandemic, and I want to say twelve, thirteen guys—maybe fourteen—laid themselves off, basically. They just said, "To hell with this shit, I'm filing for unemployment. We're not 'essential.'" But the thing is, we fell under a "manufacturer of food and beverage" clause. It was like, "Hey, if you're manufacturing stuff for food or beverage, you all keep going in to work," which was kinda strange. Because I knew a lot of construction workers who were getting laid off, and their companies were taking that step and saying, "Hey, look, we don't do no work at hospitals. We don't do no work at this place or that place. We're just gonna lay everybody off. Y'all stay safe, stay home, and whenever this shit starts to calm down we're gonna bring everybody back and pick it all back up."

So we had these guys lay themselves off, like I said. And I spoke to my wife. We talked about what to do for a good solid week there. She was able to work from home once they closed the daycares down. We got a fourteen-year-old, a ten-year-old, and a two-year-old. And our two-year-old—his daycare was done. They were shutting the doors. And so my wife told her bosses, "Look, I got to work from home." Well, she could do that. I couldn't. We talked about it, and I was like, "Look, I got a number in my head. If this shit starts killing 4,500 to 5,000 Americans a day . . . that's my line in the sand." I said, "That's when I'll become a full-on recluse. But until that point, I'm gonna continue to go to work every day. I'm gonna stay away from people, I'm gonna socially distance—the only people I'm going to be around is us." And that's the way we did it. But, man, it was like our company . . . they took it so personal. Because the guys who laid themselves off—almost all of them were frickin' studs at work. Really good coppersmiths, sheet metal mechanics, whatever you want to call 'em. Good workers. And our company got really upset when they left. They was like, "Well, if you're gonna lay yourself off, come get your tools" and this and that. "We're still working."

It was April 1 when the first COVID relief package came into effect, and that was . . . I think it was a Monday. I texted the president of the company that Sunday night, because I'm one of the union stewards at our company. We got two of us—there's another guy who's been the union steward longer. But there was some times when I needed to step in, so the union hall was like, "Look, y'all can have two stewards." That's why there are two of us. So I texted her, the president of the company, and I said, "I need to get y'all's ears tomorrow—you, your siblings, and your cousins. We need to have a talk."

Next day I go in to work and they called me up to the office around ten, and they're like, "Hey, what's going on?" I said, "Look, as of today, all of the options for working people are open." For instance, you had the Families First Coronavirus Response Act, and one of the things that did was make companies with over fifty employees, like us, eligible to receive aid to compensate for workers having to miss some time for daycare. A lot of union sheet metal companies in the city—they weren't eligible for that because they didn't have enough employees to qualify, which I always thought was crazy. Congress, I believe, dropped the ball on that one. So I told them—I said, "Look, I know you're all upset with those guys who laid themselves off, but you shouldn't be. They're just doing what's best for their families. All them guys laid themselves off because they didn't feel like this was 'essential' work. They were just listening to our politicians and our health professionals. Some of those guys have children who are at higher risk, others have family members, wives, etc. who are frontline workers in major hospitals in the city. In their minds they're thinking, 'I'm not gonna get this shit and bring it home and spread it to all these people.'"

I was trying to make them see all sides. I said, "You all need to prove to us that we are 'essential.' Because the people you have out there working right now—they're going to stick it out here and work through this, they're going to follow all the rules and all the rule changes. But there's a lot of guys out there who might not." And at that time there was about eleven more guys who were telling me, "Look, I'm not gonna sit here and continue to do this when I can make $400 a week on unemployment doing what the politicians are telling me to do. The bosses are trying to say we're 'essential.' We're not. If we were 'essential' we would be getting compensated for being 'essential.'" That was the big consensus. Because everybody was looking to me, you know? They were telling me, "Hey, this is bullshit. We're the largest contractor in this local, we're doing work for all these different places. The top dogs here at this company need to know we're not doing this."

So I went to the president and the rest of the family that owns the company and I told them that. And they said, "Look, there's interest-free loans and stuff we're looking at. We're going to give everybody a pay raise. We don't know what percentage it's going to be just yet, but everybody who's sticking with us, everybody who's still working, is gonna get something. We're gonna talk to the bank, we got a conference call with our lawyers today," etc., etc. And two weeks later they came out and said that everybody, no matter what their classification was, everybody was gonna get paid 25 percent more. They said, "Everybody's gonna get 25 percent until the governor gives the 'all-clear' for construction to go back," more or less. So, they came through and they put their money where their mouth was. And for about six or seven weeks there we got 25 percent more. That was when things were getting really bad with COVID. Those were the worst times—up to that point, at least. But we know what happened from there. More and more you saw things were opening back up around the country, then they closed back down. Then, of course, at the end of October, around Halloween, shit started hitting the fan again. They wasn't telling people to stay home like they was before. Well, in certain places around the country they were. In parts of California—in hotspots like L.A. and the whole San Joaquin Valley—they were shutting things down. So . . . it's been a roller coaster.

It was weird there for a while, you know . . . driving to work. We start work at six in the morning, and it takes me about twenty-four minutes in the morning to get to work—about twenty-seven to get home in the afternoon. And I just remember driving to work back in the spring and, like, there was *nobody* on the interstate. Driving through downtown Louisville you didn't see no cops, nothing. And usually it's packed. I remember sitting in my car thinking, "Is this right?" With the way unemployment and everything was going at that time—people were getting like an extra four hundred from the government or something—I just remember being like, "Should I really be going into work?" I mean, of course I'm gonna be as safe as can be—I'm gonna go to work, gonna do my job, I'm gonna be socially distanced, I'm not gonna sit with a big group of guys or anything. Not that I could, because our company put a lock on the frickin' breakroom. They said, "Everybody bring your own snacks, don't use the refrigerators, wash the door handles, etc." They was taking precautions. In fact, *they* was the ones buying up all the damn sanitizing wipes. I don't know how the hell they was getting them, because you couldn't get that shit in the grocery stores or anywhere at that time.

Max: Right!

Kyle: But somehow our work got boxes of those things delivered. And I was like, "How are y'all doing that? How are y'all getting that shit?" [Laughs.] But uh . . . yeah, it was all very weird. It was weird going into work. And I just kept thinking, like, "Am I right? Am I wrong?" It was a hard thing to square because I was the one who kept making the point to our company, over and over. I was the one saying, "Look, don't be upset with these guys who laid themselves off and did what they felt they needed to do to protect their families." At the same time, though, I was very stern with those guys when they would come to me like, "You're fucking wrong for going to work. You're not fucking 'essential.'" I would say to them, "You know what? My wife and I—we done discussed this. That's how I make a decision. I see what's best for my family, my kids, and for her. That's my reasoning." You know what I'm saying? But I'll tell ya, man, it was something I questioned damn near every day.

And I knew a lot of people who were off, too—there were a lot of guys whose companies laid them off. And they wanted to work. It was just . . . ugh, I dunno.

I'll never forget the eeriness of the interstates. No matter which one you jumped on to go to work, it was always like, "What the hell is going on?" Because of where my house is located, I got three options for routes to take to work and they're all within, like, a minute of each other. But no matter which one I took to get to work, there was just *nobody* on the roads. There'd be nobody in the gas station—there might be one person paying at the pump. And if I wanted to buy chewing tobacco I'd have to go in there and get it, so I might see the cashier at the gas station and that's it. If it wasn't for that, my ass would not have been going in anywhere at that time.

Max: Yeah . . . it's deeply unsettling. There's like a zombie-apocalypse kind of feeling to it all . . .

Kyle: Yes! It sounds corny as hell, but that's exactly what it was like—a zombie apocalypse. That's what it would be like if there was a zombie apocalypse. Now, obviously, if there *was* a zombie apocalypse I wouldn't be worried about fabricating metal. I'd be trying to find some shell casings and some gunpowder or something, you know?

Max: [Laughs.] Right.

Kyle: I'd be foraging for berries or some shit [laughs]. But yeah, it was . . . it was odd. There was about a two-month period there when things were really creepy. That lasted until around middle or end of May. I forget exactly when Governor Beshear said, "Alright, construction folks, you all go back to work." That's when you started seeing more cars on the road. But it was really odd there for a while. And that's something I think I'm always gonna remember—the drive into work.

Max: I can picture it in my mind—I'm just imagining how eerie that must have felt. It was those abrupt changes to the normal that made everything *real*, you know? Like, you've spent years sitting in twenty-two minutes' worth of traffic to get to work . . . then, suddenly, it's just gone.

Kyle: Exactly. Then it would only take me, like, less than nineteen minutes or so to get to work . . .

Max: This may be kind of a quick detour, but you said something earlier that I wanted to follow up on. I thought of this when you said that your company had somehow managed to procure all those sanitation wipes and stuff at a time when it was so hard for people to get them. That really struck me, because that was my first big driving-on-an-empty-interstate kind of moment in the pandemic. I wasn't driving into work or anything like that, but I remember going to the supermarket back in late winter-early spring and getting that same eerie feeling. This was in the earlier days of the pandemic, so people weren't quarantining yet, but there was a general sense of unease and people were starting to take precautions. This was right around the time when you couldn't find fucking toilet paper anywhere . . .

Kyle: Oh, yeah! That was so ridiculous.

Max: Yeah, it was! I remember asking clerks at the store if they had any hand sanitizer and they just pointed to some shelves that were entirely cleaned out. All the toilet paper was cleaned out, all the medicines were cleaned out. That was one of the first really eerie moments for me. Because, man, when you grow up in this American "land of plenty," supermarkets play a pretty important role. Their job is to *always* be fully stocked with shit—just row after row of stocked shelves—and that's kind of designed to make you think that the system will always have enough to provide for its people. When you go from that to seeing the shelves empty it gives you a real shock, like you described. That disruption of the normal was deeply unsettling, and experiencing that was what made me realize that this thing was here and it was actually happening.

People may forget this in the future, but I remember there was an interesting little subplot that emerged at that point in the pandemic. Everyone was worried about getting hand sanitizer, all the store-name brands were out, so then you had a lot of distilleries start using their equipment to "brew" sanitizer, remember?

Kyle: Oh, yeah.

Max: Were those distilleries using the equipment you guys made for them?

Kyle: Yes. The distilleries switched over to producing sanitizer for about a month or so. And it made sense, because it's the easiest thing in the world—you just take ethyl alcohol, add a little glycol to it, slap it in a bottle and say, "Don't drink this shit. Put it on your hands." It's so easy to make. Well, I guess it's not *easy* per se—there's a lot of moving parts—but when it comes to the alcohol itself just get it to 172 degrees and *boom*, it's a cash cow. I'm glad you brought that up, because *that* was the thing for me—that was what made me think, "You know what? I am 'essential.'" Because if that equipment goes down, you know, we'll be able to go out there and get it fixed, whatever the problem is, and then they'll be able to get back up and continue to make hand sanitizer.

Max: Damn! That's so cool.

Kyle: But going back to the supermarket thing really quick . . . I know you said you're from Southern California originally and you've lived in other places, but have you ever been, like, caught in a big snowstorm?

Max: Oh, yeah. I was living in Michigan before this . . .

Kyle: Okay, Michigan, there ya go—prime example. So, if people are gonna go to the stores during a snowstorm to clean something out, it's always gonna be milk and bread, right? That's what they do in Louisville, at least. If we're gonna get ten inches of snow everyone's like, "Holy shit! There's gonna be no milk and bread left!" There'll be a shitload of peanut butter, a shitload of jelly, sliced ham, and boxes of cereal, but for some reason they're taking all the milk and bread. But this time instead of milk and stuff, like you said, it was all the weird shit that was getting cleaned out: medicines, toilet paper, sanitation wipes—shit that never goes out of stock. I can't remember a time when people were so concerned with cleaning that all the cleaning shit was gone. As if there was a big surplus of asses to be wiped [laughs], so they had to take all the toilet paper . . .

Max: [Laughs.] Right.

Kyle: Even the shitty, bargain-brand toilet paper! Even the John Wayne-type toilet paper—you know, "rough, tough, and doesn't take shit off of nobody." That was gone too. And it's like, "Are you kidding me?"

Max: That's when you really see the mass psychosis at work, right? Because if you see a bunch of other people with arms full of toilet paper you're thinking, "Well, they must know something I don't. Maybe there's a toilet paper shortage." You just jump headfirst into the hysteria, then other people see you jump in, then they jump in, and so on. Hell, I can even remember feeling that myself when I saw people carrying armfuls of some particular product, like laundry detergent or something. I was like, "Oh, shit. Does that mean that product is going to be gone soon? Lemme go throw five of them in my cart." And you don't really know what you're basing any of that on! It's like part survival instinct, part FOMO [Fear of Missing Out]. You just get that fear, that deeply irrational fear. And once other people start feeding off that fear and it starts spiraling, it's like a brushfire.

Kyle: Oh, yeah. If anything, I think this country, and the planet as a whole—we've learned a lot about ourselves and where we are mentally this past year. I forget who said it years ago—it might have been George Carlin or somebody—but they said, "The person is smart. They're rational, they're fast-thinking, and this and that. People, the crowd, the masses, are stupid. They're ignorant, they're irrational, and quick to jump to conclusions."

Max: The amount of wisdom in George Carlin's stand-ups is actually kind of scary.

Kyle: Oh, definitely. He's a national treasure. There's been a lot of greats, but he's up there. I'd put him in my top five.

Max: Absolutely. George is in the top five, for sure. Well, before I let you go, man, lemme ask you something. You talked earlier about how you, as a shop steward, went to the owners of the company to talk things out when the pandemic was getting serious. I meant to ask, before we got to talking about hand sanitizer, toilet paper, and George Carlin: What did all that look like on the union side of things? What were y'all discussing at the local?

Kyle: After the stewards would talk to management we would go back to the union. I'd probably call them every other day and be like, "Hey, what's y'all's take on this? The company's wanting to do this or that. How do y'all feel about that?" Overall, though, I felt like, from our contractor to the customers, everybody was just trying to make it work. And the union was kind of there with us, like, "Hey, look, we're all in uncharted waters."

I hate to imagine what it would have been like to go through all of that and not be with the union, to not have the union just a phone call away. Because the company was kind of shitty with some of the people—not all, but some. Remember when I was talking about some of the guys laying themselves off and going on unemployment? To some of them the company was like, "Oh, yeah, no problem. Come back when you feel ready." With some of the other guys, though, they wanted them to just come get their tools and clear out. And I just remember being so frustrated and so angry that day that I loaded up my tools too. I remember backing my truck into the shop, grabbing the crane, rigging up my box, and loading up all my tools. And my foreman comes over to me like, "What are you doing?" Because I was still working—I was at work. And I told him, "I'm taking my shit with me. I'm not quitting. I'm not laying myself off. I'm going to be back tomorrow."

But I was gonna take my own tools home. I remember the union folks had come down there that day when guys who had laid themselves off were loading up their toolboxes like the company told them to. I told my foreman, "I'm loading mine up in solidarity with them, because this ain't no way to treat these guys. They're going about all this the wrong way. They need to calm down, realize it's gonna be okay, and just be support-ive." I got over $4,000 worth of tools in there—and they're *my* personal tools. I said, "You know what? I shouldn't have to have this many fucking tools. They can provide me with these tools." And since then, I have not brought any of those boxes back. I'm working out of a five-gallon bucket—I have a little handheld toolbox with maybe $500 worth of tools. That's what I've been working with ever since. My big roll-around toolbox with all the little gadgets and gizmos—to hell with that shit. I don't need it to do my job. If I have to have some specialized tools I'll go see our tool department or maintenance. But yeah, man, I couldn't imagine not having the union there when all that shit was going on . . .

I'll tell you one thing, though, and I'll close on this point: It definitely has been a breath of fresh air, because I feel like a lot of people, working people—not just at our company and around the city, but all around the world—are seeing how important they really are to the grand scheme of things. You're not just a number. You're pretty important, actually. You make the money for these companies; you get the product out there. I mean, that's why it upset our company so much when guys didn't come to work, and they kind of showed their cards in that moment. Ever since then, and now that things have kind of gotten back to normal, it's really been in the workers' favor. They know they need us to do this work, to take up these special projects and make it look perfect, and we know it too. Before the pandemic, workers might have disputes and the bosses would be like, "Well, if they want to go work for another company, let 'em. This work ain't for everybody." But now they're like, "Oh, please stay!" [Laughs.]

7. Zenei Triunfo-Cortez

My name is Zenei Triunfo-Cortez. I've been a registered nurse for over four decades, and I am president of the California Nurses Association, National Nurses Organizing Committee, and a co-president of National Nurses United.

Max: Wow, you've been doing this for a long time! I really want to learn more about you and your own path into nursing. But first, having had such a long career in nursing, and given everything we've all been through with COVID-19, I wanted to start by asking the question that I'm sure is on a lot of readers' minds: Have you ever seen anything like this? Have you had anything to compare this past year to?

Zenei: Let me start by letting you know how I got into nursing. I belong to a family of nurses. I got inspired by one of my aunts, one of my dad's sisters, who was the first nurse in the family. I saw that she was very happy with her chosen career. And when she took a leave to have a family she applied all of her nursing knowledge in raising her kids. I thought, "Oh, this is such a cool profession, and it's a very stable profession. If you are ready to go back and practice nursing, there's always a job for you there." I thought it would be a good professional track to follow, and so I did.

When I started my career things were very different. Back then patients were treated very differently than how we treat them today, in the sense that if they were sick, or if there was something that they came in for, we never discharged them until they were able to get up by themselves, able to walk around, and able to really care for themselves. Nowadays they can hardly get up before we push them out. I remember back then having one of my patients go through a simple cataract surgery. She stayed in the hospital for five days. Fast forward to now: You're barely in the hospital five hours before you're sent home. That was a change that happened over time, and I had to adjust because that was the situation. Back then people had a lot of time to bond with their doctors, because they were not rushed when they had their doctor's appointment, and they had a lot of preventative care too, which meant they did not really require a lot of hospitalizations. Nowadays people come to the hospital and they're very ill, almost close to the point of dying, and that's really very disturbing for me as a nurse.

Over time, I've seen epidemics of HIV/AIDS, H1N1, and Ebola—and over this last year, of course, the pandemic of COVID-19. It's unprecedented. Even with all the other epidemics that I've been through combined, I've never seen anything like it. I thought Ebola was the worst that I would see. But COVID-19 is much, much worse. I'm hoping that, in the remaining years of my career, I won't see anything worse than what we're seeing now. I think the difference with the other epidemics that I've experienced is that they—whoever was running the country, or whoever was in positions to make decisions—relied so much more on science and what was happening in the health care world. Unfortunately, when COVID-19 hit, that was not the case. I don't think I have to say anything more than that. The former president did not really follow science or the experts and just dismissed it like it was nothing. That's the sad part. I am still really heartbroken that I have to see this, that I have to experience the deaths of friends, acquaintances, and a lot of patients. That's very disturbing for me.

It's mind-boggling that we—myself and other nurses, other health care workers, and other essential workers—would have to risk our lives because of the reckless decisions of the people who are in positions of power. Those people should have made quick decisions that could have helped us save the world, and save other health care and essential workers, but they did not do that. And so, because of that, I am really still heartbroken and very disturbed.

Max: My God, I can only imagine. Of course, we've all experienced the COVID-19 pandemic in our own ways, we've all been part of this, but so much of the cost of those decisions that were made or not made, so much of the human weight . . . all the deaths of family members, neighbors, patients . . . so much of that falls on the shoulders of you and your coworkers. For the rest of us, we only see that cost when it touches people in our circles, but for you and your fellow hospital workers it's always there, right in front of you. It's all concentrated in the place where you work. It's a day-to-day reality. I can't even begin to imagine the sheer psychological and emotional toll it has taken on you just getting through this year.

Zenei: When we learned that there was this very vile virus going around, as the leaders of our organization, we got together with our allies and other nursing groups all over the world. We all belong to Global Nurses United. At the very beginning, way back in January 2020, we crafted a letter together to ask the World Health Organization to look at this virus and give us the guidance and standards we needed so that we could stop transmission and mitigate the spread. But, unfortunately, that fell on deaf ears. Then each of the groups also wrote to their respective government agencies and presidents to encourage each country to do whatever they could. But again, here in the United States, we had a president who unfortunately did not listen to what a women-dominated profession had to say. We were dismissed, we were ignored. In the end, that took a toll on the lives of a lot of nurses and health care workers.

As nurses, we know how to follow infection-control protocols. And so we said, "Okay, if a patient is sick and we don't know what kind of virus that patient has, it would be incumbent upon us to start wearing masks and start protecting ourselves." At that time, though, a lot of our nurses were disciplined for wearing masks because hospital administration said that we were only "increasing the anxiety" of our patients. What that revealed to us was that the hospital industry was willing to kill their staff . . . that was a really heavy burden for us to carry. We would walk around the hospital with masks in our pockets, and if we didn't have any supervisor or manager around we'd put on the mask. Then, when we'd see them coming we would take it off. But we should not have had to do that. We were protecting ourselves, because we want to protect our patients—all our patients. And at the end of the day we go home to our families. We need to protect them as well. But the hospital industry didn't care, nobody cared. So, we started fighting back for ourselves and for our own protection, and for the protection of our patients. We did a lot of actions in our facilities, we did a lot of media interviews. We were out there saying to the public, "Hey, you need to support us, because we are trying to keep you all alive." Eventually, over that long period of time, we got some masks, but they were not the right kind of mask we needed, so we had to keep fighting and keep pushing for optimal protections. By the same token, the CDC [Centers for Disease Control and Prevention] were very slow with putting out their guidelines, and the hospital industry liked that, because the lack of guidelines meant they weren't obligated to protect the nurses and other health care workers. It was very, very sad.

With each COVID surge—the first wave, second wave, third wave, etc.—we lost a lot of nurses. As nurses, we made a pledge to take care of our patients no matter what, under whatever circumstances, to the point that when we rush to respond to an emergency we sometimes forget to gown up, which could lead to a nurse getting infected himself or herself and even dying. And that happened to a lot of our nurses. Then there's the issue of cross-contamination. Management came up with the decision that only nurses who are taking care of COVID patients should wear personal protective equipment. We understood that decision, but then you would have situations where those nurses would come out of a COVID-19 patient's hospital room and they'd interact with those of us who were not taking care of COVID-positive patients, so we cross-contaminated ourselves. It took a lot of our energy, a lot of our time, and a lot of our sanity to continue to fight for the optimum PPE for all of us who are working in the hospital.

It's been a very long year, and a lot of our nurses are very tired and overwhelmed—not just physically but emotionally, mentally. It's really taken a toll on us these past fourteen months. I've heard a lot of nurses who are retiring prematurely because of what's going on. I just feel sorry for the younger ones who cannot take that option. Again, first and foremost, we are here for our patients. But where do we draw the line? Do we stop because we continue to endanger our lives? Or do we keep going? We have signed up for this profession, but—and I know you've heard this before—we didn't sign up to die.

Max: I mean, we *saw* how all of this played out, and I hope that people who read this book in the future are able to recall it for themselves. During the COVID-19 pandemic, especially in the early days, there was a lot of public celebration of frontline workers, including hospital workers. There were so many commercials and billboards, so many people banging pots and pans on their balconies, etc. I really do believe a lot of people felt genuine support and gratitude for these workers. At the same time, it was like we, as a society, were just pushing these workers into the firing line without protecting them. We were basically celebrating them for dying unnecessarily, making ourselves feel better about their "sacrifice" without doing what needed to be done to protect workers like yourself who were trying to save as many lives as you possibly could. I think that really is one of the great stains that will be left on our souls from this past year. When we needed to be there for the people who were there for us, we weren't. There's really no other way to put that.

I wanted to circle back to something you said, Zenei, because I think it's really important and helps us understand how we ended up here. You mentioned that, back when you started working as a nurse, you had way more time and care and attention to give to each patient—people weren't just being cycled in and out like they were customers at a McDonald's. Now that has all changed. I wanted to ask if that was one of the original reasons you got invested in the profession. Was there something about being able to provide that type of intimate care that made you want to be a nurse? And could you talk a little bit more about how the broad changes in the hospital industry over the years contributed to making the situation with COVID worse, especially here in the United States.

Zenei: What really drew me into this profession is the fact that I'm a people person and, you know, I want to help people, whether they're my friend, an acquaintance, or I don't know them at all. I thought nursing would be the profession that would allow me to help people, especially when they're in their most vulnerable situations.

When I started nursing I would spend as much time as I could with a patient. I remember being there holding a patient's hand when the doctor told them they had cancer, staying with the patient as long as I could to help alleviate their anxiety. I also remember talking to the family when they'd come to visit, explaining everything to them, and kind of being part of their family as well. That really was a fulfilling time for me back then. As time evolved, health care became an industry, a corporation, and everything changed. They started to set goals like, "If you're having your appendix removed, you can only be in the hospital for X amount of days, and you're only allowed this amount of time in nursing, this amount of time in the operating room, etc."—kind of like a one-size-fits-all approach. And our professional judgment as nurses, I thought, would eventually be ignored, because it wouldn't matter what I had to say—everything would have to follow the recipe handed down from the hospital industry. But that's not how it should be, because patients are individuals and they have individual needs. If we just follow the direction of the hospital industry it would be like, "Oh, if you're having your appendix removed, you're only required to be here an hour, and no matter what situation you are in, after an hour you're out of here." And the bed that patient just vacated? It's still warm, and they want to put another patient in it. If you're an old-school nurse, that bothered you, because that's not how we were trained, that's not how we were educated in school, but we needed to adapt because that was the situation, and it just got worse over time. It's kind of like an assembly line, if I may say, and it's not right, because our patients are human beings and we need to treat them with respect. We need to be more compassionate. Nurses still have that compassion, I don't doubt that. But the people in the hospital industry who are making these decisions do not see that. They're not there at patients' bedsides. They're not there in the patient care areas. They're in their offices crunching numbers, making sure they get their bottom line, their profits, even though they say they're a "not-for-profit" institution. It's their excess revenue, I would say, that they are really occupied with—they want to make sure they have a lot of that.

It's a lot of work for us, then, because we're not only fighting for the rights of our patients, we're fighting for our rights as well. It's a lot to take on, and I admire my colleagues for taking on whatever challenge we're faced with on any given day. I sure hope the public realizes that. Actually, I know they do, because nursing has been voted the most trusted profession for many years in a row. But I just want the people who are making the decisions for us to realize that their business is about taking care of human lives. And the people doing the work that makes that business run are human beings as well. We get tired, we get burnt out, and we need breaks. They need to realize that.

You mentioned the celebrations over the last year. There were a lot of people calling us heroes. There was an endless delivery of food, billboard signs, lawn signs, etc. As much as I appreciated the accolades and the gestures, we didn't need that. What we needed was PPE. We could have avoided the deaths of many more nurses if, instead of spending money on publicity and marketing saying how much nurses and other health care workers are appreciated, hospitals channeled that money into buying or acquiring the PPE we were asking for and providing us with the additional staff that was so badly needed. From outside of the hospital, what everybody saw was, "They love their nurses! They love their health care workers! Just look at the billboard." And yet, within the hospital walls, nurses and health care workers were struggling . . . we were struggling.

Each day I walked into the hospital I never knew what kind of day I was going to have. I never knew if I would be provided with an N95 mask—that was the minimum PPE I could have—or if I would be able to get a gown to protect me, or head and shoe covers. I never knew if I would get those basic things. Then it came to a point when they said, "We do not have enough N95s to last us throughout the course of the pandemic because we don't know when it's going to end." So they asked us to reuse our N95s for as long as we could. But it's a single-use mask and we need to dispose of it after each encounter with a patient. But because we were using it for patient A, for patient B, for patient C, in our minds we were cross-contaminating among those patients. We tried our best to wipe it down, even though you're not supposed to use alcohol to wipe it down, and do whatever we could. Then the hospital industry came up with another idea: All of the masks should go into one bin, then they would use a decontamination method where the masks would go through a chemical process, then they would be given back to us for use. We were inhaling chemicals because we were being asked to reuse those decontaminated masks. And yet, we still came to work. When we were with a patient we were calm and professional like, "Nothing wrong is happening, we're here to take care of you. We will take care of you, we will help you get well." But within us, on the inside, we were struggling, because we're using a decontaminated mask, it's giving us headaches, it's giving us migraines, we don't know what the long-term effects might be. Yet we continued to do our work.

Max: You already started to talk about this, but I just wanted to drill down on it so that readers can really understand what it was like for you and your coworkers this past year. Like you were saying, most of us only saw things from the outside. We saw the billboards from hospitals saying, "We love our nurses" and all that stuff. But inside there was so much pain, so much struggle, so much burnout that people weren't seeing. I know there was no such thing as a "typical workday" during COVID-19, but do you think you could just paint a picture of what it was like to walk through the hospital doors around this time last year, when the first wave was really kicking off and things were getting really bad? From the moment you walked in for a shift to the moment you walked out, what sort of things were you being asked to do?

Zenei: Coming to work during this time last year, when we were hitting the surge, I never knew what was going to happen. But we continued to work and we continued to come to work. We continued to take on our assignments and we did what we needed to do. But deep inside me there was a lot of fear. "Will I be contaminating myself? Will I get the virus?" Then, at the end of the day, "Am I going home to my family with the virus?"

A lot of our nurses have young kids, and there's always that fear of bringing the virus home, and of interacting with the public. You stop by the grocery store to perhaps pick up a gallon of milk for the kids, but the whole time you're thinking, "Am I contaminating the people around me in the grocery store?" And then you come home. Some of us live in multigenerational households where we have our parents in the house, and we might have some family members who are immunocompromised, so that has always been a source of our fear. Fortunately for me it's just me and my husband here in the house, but you still think about the exposure you've had at work. Then I would visit my immunocompromised sister, but I would always make sure that I'd come home first, strip down, take a shower, etc. But you're always worrying, "Is the virus still there? Did I wash up enough? Did I shower enough?" Again, because we did not have adequate PPE needed to protect ourselves in the work environment, you don't know if somewhere in your body you are carrying it—that was enough to keep you awake at night. Then you'd only have a couple of hours of sleep before you'd go back to work. Walking into the hospital you're wondering,

"Will I have an N95? A *fresh* N95? Will I have gowns? Will I have a head cover? Will I have shoe covers? How will my patients be doing today? Will I lose another patient? Will I be able to set up a FaceTime call between my patients and their families?" Those are the kinds of things that keep going through your mind day in, day out. And no two days are the same, because there will be days when a patient is doing well, but then there will be days when other patients will crash and require more care and more of your time—and in the back of your mind you know you still have other patients waiting for you.

We did not have enough staff to carry out a full shift, and we didn't have enough reserves to fill in. Our coworkers were getting sick, a lot of them had taken medical leave. So you're dealing with that, and you're seeing it happening right in front of you, and it's very hard. All the while, in the back of my mind, I'm thinking of a very good friend who is the charge nurse (a lead nurse who is in charge or oversees a specific unit) at a different hospital who contracted the virus and is on a ventilator—and she's very young. Then you hear about a former coworker who was found dead in her apartment. She was here in California and moved to New York, and when her coworkers did a wellness check they found her dead. Then you hear about other acquaintances who have gotten the virus and have been placed on a ventilator. And you hear about how they're running out of ventilators. So, all of those things are playing in your mind every day. But you need to kind of put it in the back of your mind, because you are dealing with your own situation at the hospital: taking care of your patient, fighting for your PPE, and basically fighting for your own life as well. For me, professionally, I know what to do, because these are infection control protocols that I learned in school and that I have practiced throughout my career. However, at this moment, in this time of COVID, I am being told to not follow what I know and to bypass a lot of steps. I know it's bad because that's not what my practice has been, that's not what I was taught in school. It's morally distressing, it's physically distressing, and it's mentally distressing. It was too much.

Max: I think you said it all: that is too much to ask of anyone. Of course, this has been a situation that we couldn't completely control. A pandemic is certainly what an insurance company would call an "act of God," right?

It's a terrible thing, it happened, and we had to deal with it as best we could. What I hope is getting through to readers, though, is that there were so many ways we could have made it *less* terrible. There were so many deaths that we could have prevented but didn't. Obviously, workers in places like hospitals were always going to bear the brunt of something like COVID-19, but like you were saying, there's still so much that you and your coworkers shouldn't have had to deal with.

That actually brings me to a question I wanted to ask you, Zenei, but only if you're comfortable talking about it. As we look back at the devastation of the past year, there are things that we need to sit with, think about, and learn from. We need to ask ourselves, "Why did this happen the way it did? Could it have been different? Could we have done better? Could we have prevented more of these unbearable deaths? And why were some people hit harder than others?" For instance, I think the statistic that really sticks out to me is that, as of this month, 25 percent of registered nurses who have died of COVID-19 in the U.S. were of Filipino descent. That blows my mind! I wanted to ask you about that statistic and how it might also connect to the fact that the political atmosphere surrounding COVID-19, especially here in the U.S., was very much shaped by this pervasive, racist, anti-Asian fear. We saw so many examples of people being assaulted on the street, people having things yelled at them, people facing death threats. Did you see or experience any of this yourself? And why were Filipino nurses so overrepresented in the death counts even though they only make up around 4 percent of the nursing workforce?

Zenei: Let me say just a little bit more about what we did in order to stop or to mitigate the deaths. At the height of the pandemic, when we were fighting for PPE and so much more, we wanted to do it for all nurses and health care workers. Remember when I told you that they were asking us to use the decontaminated masks that had gone through the chemical process? Well, we had to prove to them that it was causing a lot of headaches and migraines and causing the nurses to be ill. We told them, "If you want us to continue using these masks, this is what's going to happen: you're going to lose nurses, you're going to lose health care workers." With our massive campaign, though, we were able to stop that—at least we were able to fight that off, and we were able to win it for all of us. Then the hospital came up with another idea. Here in California we have a set nurse-to-patient ratio. If you're a nurse working in the medical surgical area you only have up to five patients. So here I am, struggling with my five patients, because my patients are sicker and require more care, but that did not stop the hospital from applying for waivers to circumvent the ratios. How can they even think about that? They even told the governor, "Hey, because we are so short-staffed, the nurses should not have a limit of five." It all goes back to my point about how these people making the decisions are not there to see the reality on the ground. And so, we had to fight—we had to fight that waiver, because every hospital in this state, and in every other place you can imagine, rallied their state governments to say that nurses need to have more patients. We *already have* a lot of patients, but that's not the point. We need more *time* for our patients, which means we need fewer patients.

Last year, during the month of May, we had National Nurses' Week. It's the week to celebrate nurses, so we got a lot of accolades, a lot of recognition, a lot of fanfare, but what we needed was the PPE, and we needed more staff, and we needed safer working conditions. But that was all ignored and drowned out by the public celebration of nurses outside of the hospital walls. It's 2021 now and a lot of our nurses around the country are still fighting for the PPE they need. We have wanted the CDC and the Occupational Safety and Health Administration [OSHA] to issue an emergency temporary standard saying that COVID-19 is transmitted by aerosol . . . you can inhale it. We wanted them to recognize that so that they can give us strong guidance that our hospital employers will be mandated to follow, which would include giving us better protection. We need more than N95 masks—the N95 is just the minimum. We're also demanding the emergency temporary standard from OSHA because it's essential that we have it not just to protect nurses and health care workers, but all essential workers as well. The people who prepare our food, who work in the processing plants—all that work is essential, and we need all the protection we can get in order to stop the spread and mitigate the transmission. But guess how they celebrated the nurses instead? They took away a standard that was helping us mitigate the transmission of COVID-19. According to the CDC, you do not have to wear a mask if you're fully vaccinated, but only 37 percent of adults in our country are fully vaccinated right now. Instead of giving us more protection they took away another layer of protection that's helping us and that's helping protect the public. The CDC says, "If you're fully vaccinated, you can go out, mingle without a mask, go celebrate without a mask, and the people around you don't have to wear a mask if they're fully vaccinated." But how do I know that you're fully vaccinated? How do I know this person on my right or the person on my left is fully vaccinated?

Every day roughly six hundred people continue to die of COVID-19 in the U.S.[7] Our nurses continue to die. We continue to have high numbers of COVID-infected patients. So why are they doing that? Why is the CDC saying this? They say the decision is based on studies—what studies? They were citing studies that were done in a different country—I think it was Israel—but studies have different benchmarks, and we need to look at what the science is telling us is happening here in the U.S. We need to be precise. We are fighting now to have the CDC revoke their decision for the unmasking of fully vaccinated people. As always, it's a struggle, it's a fight. But we will continue to fight because we are here not just for our patients in the hospital, but we're here for the health and welfare of the public. And it's going to be a public health crisis if there's another surge in COVID-19 cases. Along with our everyday struggles at the bedside, then, we were also fighting on a much larger scale. If it's not one thing it's another. But we were able to fight back that nurse-to-patient ratio waver and that was a big win for us. I'm so glad we have a strong union that supports us, that unites all of the nurses so we can fight on a larger scale.

However, in spite of fighting all these fights—and winning most of them—our nurses continued to die. And more so with Filipino-American nurses. Why is that? Well, I'm Filipino and I can tell you that, among other things, we have been labeled as being hungry for money, even during this time when we are fighting COVID and fighting for our lives. They said, "Oh, yeah, a lot of them have died because they're so money-hungry, they're doing a lot of overtime," etc. But that's not the reason why Filipino-American nurses stay for long hours. Culturally, we treat our patients like they are our families. If a manager or a supervisor comes to me and says, "Can you stay? There's nobody who can work," that translates to, "There

7 This interview took place on May 24, 2021.

will be no nurse for your patients." What do I say to that? I don't want it on my conscience that I deliberately left the hospital knowing that there would be no nurse for X amount of patients. So we tend to stay. That is one of the reasons why a lot of the Filipino nurses have died. On top of that, Filipino-American nurses tend to work in the critical care areas where COVID-19 patients are being cared for—in intensive care units, in the telemetry units where patients are monitored—and people working in those areas took a big hit. Even though we only make up 4 percent of the workforce, we are in the areas where the COVID patients are housed in the hospital. The other thing, too, is that we tend to overlook our own welfare in order to look out for the welfare of the group. Some of our Filipino-American nurses have responded to an emergency without putting on the PPE because they wanted to save the patient's life. They overlooked their own welfare. And so, again, all of these things took a toll on Filipino-American nurses.

When the pandemic hit and President Trump was still in office he labeled the virus as the "Chinese virus," and there were also some assertions from other people in government who said it was a lab-manufactured virus that originated in China, so on and so forth. A lot of Asians were targeted, and it kind of escalated because we were being blamed for what was going on. And I think a lot of folks cannot distinguish Chinese from Filipinos from Thailanders from Vietnamese, so we were all just labeled as "Asians." It's very disappointing that, instead of objecting to the rumors and the mislabeling, we had a president who perpetuated hate and racism. I know for a fact that racism has been institutionalized in many places, but it has also been perpetuated and reinforced by a president who is out of his mind, I would say. And it's very heartbreaking because, again, as a Filipina, as an Asian, you want to do what's good, you want to do what's right, and yet there are forces out there who dislike you, who hate you. Even if you tend to do good and you tend to do right for them, you're still the Asian, you're still the person from Asia, where the virus came from. "We don't like you here. You should go back to your country. You should go back to where you belong." It often comes in subtle ways. I have been in situations where there were subtle insinuations that were like, "Hey, you're Asian—go back to where you belong. You don't deserve this country." But I tend to ignore it, you know? I just kind of let it go. But in some of the cases with our nurses it's been more obvious and more pronounced. We had a labor and delivery nurse who was helping a patient deliver and then the husband—obviously, they're Caucasian—came out and said, "I want a White nurse to help my wife!" But the response from the nurse was, "Well, in that case, you will be helping your wife, because there are no other nurses except Asians or nurses of color." The husband didn't say anything after that and just allowed the nurse to help his wife. Maybe it happens every day and we just tend to play it down and dismiss it—we don't want to make a big deal out of it. But we carry it every day, we carry it in our minds and in our hearts. And it's . . . I am beyond words, really, because it has never been so blown up, so brazen. We need to end it.

There's one more thing I would say, though, while we're on the subject. The health disparity between people of color—Black, Indigenous, Latinx—and White people has always been pronounced, mainly because of the health care system that we have, but that disparity just became more apparent with this pandemic. If you're working the tendency is that you have some kind of health care, but with COVID a lot of people got laid off, a lot of people lost their jobs, and then they lost their health care coverage. That created a whole new world of problems, because now we have this pandemic *and* people do not have access to health care. But if we had a Medicare for All system, the single-payer system that we have been fighting for for so many years, then we would not have this problem. People could get the health care they need when they need it, because it wouldn't be tied to their jobs, which would also mean that they can always seek better paying jobs and better working conditions without the threat of losing health care coverage. And if that were the case there wouldn't be as much discrimination. Because right now, if you come to the hospital, we can see if your insurance is under public aid. I'm not saying that the health care workers would discriminate against you, but patients do have that feeling that they will not be given the same level of care as somebody who has better insurance. Medicare for All would eliminate all of that stigma, that feeling of not being able to get better care or better treatment—that would all go away. And we *want* that to go away, obviously. That's why we're fighting for single-payer.

Going back to the racist attacks on Asians, our union has issued a statement condemning those attacks. A lot of our nurses spoke out about the racist attacks on Asians, as well as the racism against Black people. We also have statements supporting the Black Lives Matter movement. Again, it's just too much to watch every day, which is why our nurses are not just focused on health care—we're focused on a lot of other social justice issues as well. It's a bigger fight, and it's a constant fight. My dream is that in the future, and in the near future, we will have a Medicare for All system, a system that brings everybody in and leaves nobody out, so we can finally have equity in health care. We will also eliminate the disparities we've seen in the distribution of and access to COVID tests and vaccines. And there *is* a big disparity, and it's . . . it's just too much. There are too many things in our system that need to be fixed. But it's our life, and we continue to fight every day.

8. Rick "Redman" Norman

My name's Rick Norman. I'm sixty-four years old, about two months away from being on Medicare. So I guess that would be a real, legitimate *old*. I grew up in the panhandle of North Idaho—basically a very small town, about a population of four hundred, called Clark Fork, up by the Pend Oreille Lake. It was a little logging town. I don't know if you'd call it middle class. I'd call it the lower end of middle class cuz we were pretty damn poor, but everybody else was too, so I guess we didn't know it. But it was kind of like *Mayberry R.F.D.* Everybody got together and we made our own little baseball diamonds and hooked up and went fishing together, played baseball and basketball together, and everybody's mother was *everybody's* mother. They told us when it was time to go home—well, generally, when the old streetlights come on you'd go home. We talk about it all the time, how lucky we were to grow up in a small town like that. We didn't have a lot of influences, besides our parents just telling us what to do.

As hard as our parents worked—my dad worked in the sawmill and Mom was a cook at the local restaurant—the wages weren't big. We just didn't have money, you know? But in a lot of ways it was good, because we knew that *we* had to make money to get school clothes. Us kids, I mean. I delivered papers. Hell, I had two paper routes at the same time, at the *Spokane Chronicle* and the *Spokesman-Review*, both out of Spokane, Washington. I'd deliver one in the morning, then I'd have the other one in the evening. Besides that I mowed lawns, and all that money went to school clothes. So it wasn't like I was spoiled. I was the youngest of the kids: Mom had two families. My dad was her second husband, but she raised five kids on her own after she divorced her first husband. Then, when she got married to my dad, she raised three more kids. Of course, being a cook, she knew how to cook, and when she cooked a pot of spaghetti we ate spaghetti for three or four days until it was gone. That's just the way we lived our life. I don't know how much more cookie-cutter it could get.

Anyways, that's the way I grew up. I think I learned a lot about saving money. I learned a lot about work ethic. My dad was a good worker and all, but he had a bit of a temper. He would get fired from one job then go to another job and get fired again. The way he told it to me was that he was always sticking his nose into somebody else's business—like if a boss was picking on somebody, he'd go chew the boss out and then he'd get fired. We ended up moving down to southern Idaho at one point, after I went through grade school there in Clark Fork, and he went to work in a ball mill at a silver mine in Clayton, Idaho. That's down by the Salmon River. And Mom told him then, "This is it. You don't hold onto this job, we're done." This is stuff I learned later on—I didn't know none of this was going on when I was growing up.

I went to high school down there, and I ended up working in that ball mill with Dad in the summers. I also did some dishwashing at the cafe that Mom worked at down there. I was always working, always saving, always learning about the pride of making your own money. And I still have that same mindset. In fact, I'm married to a woman who, when I first met her . . . she was talking about going shopping. "Let's go shopping," she said. I go, "Okay, for what?" She said, "I don't know, just shopping, looking for deals." *"Are you out of your mind?"*

Max: [Laughs.]

Rick: I never shopped in my life unless I had a list of things I needed. And you don't deviate from that list, because you're on a budget. She's basically still that way [laughs]. All she needs is that credit card and she's happy. She's not as strict as I am about it. But anyways, we get by.

Max: I mean, you say she's not as strict as you . . . doesn't sound like it's too hard to not be that strict. [Laughs.]

Rick: Well, it isn't. She's just loose with it, and I'm probably tight. There's some middle ground there. We've been married since '85, so I guess it works.

Max: Damn, that's great! Congratulations, man.

Rick: Yeah. Once you get past the part where you're good looking and you're too old and ugly to find another one, you better just stick with what you've got and be happy. [Laughs.]

Max: [Laughs.]

Rick: I think that's the secret to a long, happy marriage.

Max: There's wisdom in that for sure [laughs]. It's so amazing to hear all of this. I know you said that it couldn't get much more cookie-cutter than the life you had growing up, but I'm just transfixed by it, because it's so different from how I grew up. I was raised in Southern California, where there are streets and cars from the ocean all the way to the mountains. So growing up in a town with a population of four hundred is very much the *opposite* of cookie-cutter for me. But I could just see it in my head as you were talking about it. When you were describing how the streetlamps would come on, how everybody's mom was everybody's mom, it just painted such a vivid picture for me. And that was in Clark Fork, right? Where did you guys go when you moved to southern Idaho?

Rick: That was down in Clayton, Idaho. And that was a population of twenty-seven at the time.

Max: Oh, wow! I was about to ask what southern Idaho was like in the late '60s and early '70s. But I guess if you have a population of twenty-seven there are only so many things that it can be. [Laughs.]

Rick: Well, down in that country, it's beef country. It's cattle ranches, high-school rodeos—you know, redneck. I was never a cowboy, but I had a lot of friends who were. And those kids . . . they were tough. Some of them, I went out and stayed on their ranches—they were friends of mine. And they had to wake up before the school bus got there to do their chores. You talk about a work ethic, man . . . they're out there doing all that stuff, then washing up and catching the bus to school. They've got in some good work before the bell even rings. I never was into that, but I would go out there and have them sourdough pancakes and some of the biggest breakfasts I've ever seen, because they also had ranch hands helping them irrigate the fields and moving sprinkler pipe, etc.

I did a lot of horseback riding, though. I love that, man. I miss it so much. They had old Indian caves up in the rocky hillsides overlooking the Salmon River, and we would go up in those old caves and find arrowheads and markings on the walls and stuff. This is all sagebrush, antelope coun-try—things only grow if you irrigated it. But ranching was never part of my life. I wasn't into that, but I was amazed by it. And those kids—boy, they grew up tough. They grew up with muscles on them and they weren't timid. And like I said, they had the high-school rodeo. Their dads would make those little fifty-gallon barrels with the cables coming off of them so the little kids could get on there and get used to bucking and bull riding. Then, by the time they're in high school, they're in the rodeo. It was a life-style that was far from Clark Fork in North Idaho—that was more logging country, so it was a whole different life.

After high school I came back up north, got married, and started work-ing here in Wallace, Idaho. So I know lots of people in lots of places, and none of them are the same. The music they listen to is different, the life-style is different—just different people. And their views on life—I didn't know what the hell they were then, but now you get on Facebook and find a lot of these people. I didn't have an inch of political awareness at all when I was young, but now I can think back and, yeah, that was a conser-vative bunch down there in southern Idaho, and I understand why. It's just different everywhere you go, you know? But the work ethic is the same. They had livings to make, and they worked hard. To my estimation, there's nobody that works harder than a farmer or rancher, because it's sunup to sundown, as hard as they can go, and it's something different every day. There's just no time for vacation. It's just unbelievable what they have to do to make a living that way.

Max: Mmhmm.

Rick: But most of them grew up that way. And they don't know a hell of a lot different, I don't think.

Max: It's wild to think about, man. I'm putting myself back into my high-school shoes and I'm thinking about all the mental preparation that went into getting ready for that week's varsity basketball game or something like that. I'd be training, I'd go running, I'd be shooting hoops until sundown and thinking about the school we were gonna play . . . I can't imagine how I would prepare if I knew that I was going to be playing a team full of ranchers and cowboys who are working their asses off from four in the morning till night. [Laughs.]

Rick: I'll tell ya, it wasn't so bad in basketball, but in football? These boys hit *hard*. And I was just a skinny little shit. Hell, I still am. I'm like 185 pounds and six-three. So you can imagine what I was in high school. I wasn't a top athlete. At best I was average, but I loved to play. I just loved it. But I'm telling you what, them boys from Mackay and southern Idaho . . . Arco, Sugar City, Salem . . . they were tough customers, boy. To this day I think that's the hardest I've ever been hit. I remember running back to the huddle and I could barely make out where my teammates were. There was just a little bit of light at the end of my tunnel. And as soon as I got back to the huddle, they clapped their hands and said, "Break!" I didn't have a clue what the goddamn play was, but I was a wide receiver, and I ran out there hoping that it wasn't going to come to me. [Laughs.]

Max: [Laughs.]

Rick: They were tough boys. It was pretty impressive. And a lot of them to this day are still running their ranches, their dad's ranches, the same piece of ground, just getting it done. I would just love to go back and see some of them. I see their faces on Facebook today and there's a small resemblance to the way I remember them, but I almost got to go back to my high school yearbook to remember what they looked like when they were little. Most of them put on a lot more weight than I did [laughs]. I stayed skinny. They're gonna know me right off the bat.

Max: [Laughs.] Yeah, you're definitely the exception that proves the rule on that front. I hope you get to see them again, though. It's so interesting to think about people like the ones you knew growing up, folks who are still working their parents' farms and stuff like that. Did you have a sense of what you wanted to grow up to do? Because I imagine, for a lot of these farming kids, it was kind of a given what they were going to do . . .

Rick: Yeah. I can tell you, I was in awe of those guys, because they did have their futures kind of set. But you could tell even then that they love that lifestyle. Their way of having fun was going to the rodeo, whether they were a participant or in the audience watching. As for me, my dreams, really, as far back as I could remember—they were always about sports. And I didn't have a shot in hell at it, but that's what my dreams were. I started on our basketball team—we had a not very good basketball team, but I started on it. So, it wasn't like I was terrible, but it wasn't a dream fulfilled. Let's put it that way. Other than that, I just wanted to have fun and make money. The dreams never really got realistic until I was probably in my mid-twenties. Then my dreams were just, you know, not die, for one thing, because I partied pretty hard during my early twenties, and I escaped death a few times. And just get married, settle down, have my own house and wife and kids. I'm back to the cookie-cutter thing there . . . But, man, sometimes that's just an achievement in itself, just to have the white picket fence thing. And that's basically where I'm at right now with my retirement that I've saved all my life, and I'm pretty happy with where I'm at.

Max: That's great, man. Like you said, that ain't nothing to be ashamed of. I know you said you're talking to me right now in your gun room and you got your fishing poles, you got your books—I'm envious, man. I can only hope to have that setup when I retire . . . if I retire. I assume it was when you went back up to North Idaho that you got into mining?

Rick: Well, after I graduated high school I came back up to North Idaho, basically to hook up with my old buddies that I left in grade school—the ones I grew up with. I went to college up there, and that lasted about half a semester. Then my dad had a stroke and I kind of used that as an excuse to drop out. Bad mistake . . . Anyways, I dropped out and kind of did the hippie scene for a year or two, worked in a sawmill, and then I came over here to Wallace because a buddy of mine was over here. I ended up getting a job at the Bunker Hill zinc plant. Let's see . . . that was November of '76. I started there and worked there for a couple years, then I pulled one of my dad's moves and had a little argument with a boss and I got fired. I ended up going into the mine after that. But the union from Bunker Hill was strong back then, and they called me up after I started working at that other mine and said, "We got your job back." And I thought, "Well, I was only making like $16,000 a year back in '77 and they were making $40,000 a year in this mine. The actual miners, that is—the drill blast guys. So there was no way I was gonna go back to Bunker Hill. But it was amazing that they got my job back because, I mean, I *should* have been fired. I kicked the door down.

Max: [Laughs.]

Rick: I was kind of hotheaded, but this guy deserved it. Anyways, I got fired, and I should have been fired. It was a good move in the end, though, because I started making a lot better money. That's how I ended up in the mines. Bunker Hill didn't last a hell of a lot longer—they shut down about three years after that. That whole zinc plant and the lead smelter—that all got torn down. Then the EPA came in and did a big cleanup all through this valley, and the rest is history.

Max: I was curious to ask more about this—and this is really more my own ignorance than anything—because when I think of Idaho I think of what you were describing before: the cowboys, the farming, etc. I guess, growing up, I just didn't know a whole lot about how much mining was going on in Idaho. Is it a pretty big industry in parts of Idaho?

Rick: Right here in Wallace, they call this the Silver Valley. They used to call it the Coeur d'Alene Mining District. Now, I'm not a geologist, but I'll give you a kind of a view of what it looks like in this country right here. It's kind of like when you have choppy water out on a lake. You get all these little peaks, like, just a crapload of peaks—this country is like that. It's almost like pyramid mountains—they all come to sharp points at the top, and they're just all over. In between those mountains are creeks and little draws, and almost every one of those little draws has either a prospecting hole or an actual old mine from the late 1800s and early 1900s. There were hundreds of mines in a small little area in this valley here. See, we're right up next to the Montana border, and then it goes west from there. This valley is, I'm going to say, thirty or thirty-five miles long, and there's just all kinds of ore here.

They originally discovered gold just a little bit north of here, probably not more than ten miles north from Wallace as the crow flies. They had placer gold up there, and that's got its own history. Then when that kind of played out—that didn't last too many years—they kind of trickled down south here to this valley and started discovering silver and lead outcroppings. They'd just see them right out there on the surface, stake a claim, and start mining. And this is back in the donkey days where an old prospector had to go up and chip away and work their asses off with no air drills, or water, or anything. Everything was dry drillin' and old candle lights—it was rough, hardcore work. But there was just all kinds of claims, and some claims hit it big. And I mean really big. There were lots of millionaires came out of this country.

Then the mining companies started consolidating and getting their little mine-owner organizations together, and a lot of these little draws became the places for several different mines. Then they got a railway going right through there at the bottom of these canyons. And, like I say, these mountains are so close together, so the railway would be right on the road. Then you would have houses trying to squeeze their way in there, and you got snow slides coming down and wiping out houses. It was just crazy. They had entire towns just stuck together so close in the bottom of these little draws that, when the train come, they would have to roll up the awnings like a bar, or a drugstore, or whatever to give room for the train to come through, get the concentrates from the mills, and then ship them out. These were wild days. These miners worked hard and played hard, and this place has a history.

Even when I was mining there . . . I started in March of '79 . . . Wallace was pretty wild. You'd go downtown on a Friday or Saturday night and it was wild. Too wild for me—I got my ass kicked in Wallace [laughs]. I had to go down to Kellogg, which was about twenty miles away, down with the Bunker Hill boys. I knew more people there. I was kind of unknown up here. So, you know, you come in here and everybody wants to test your water. But they had all kinds of whorehouses in Wallace. I'm gonna say five different whorehouses at least. One of them is a museum now, and another one they made into a melodrama thing that they do. It's kind of a tourist thing, but they have an old, Snidely Whiplash type of melodrama that they do during the summers at this old bordello. See, the whole town is a historical monument, so they have all these old buildings and houses that get funded to keep up their original look. This town basically looks the same as it did in the early 1900s. And it was wild and wooly until, I'm gonna say, around 1991, when the FBI come in and shut down all the whorehouses and took all the slot machines. All the backroom gambling stopped . . . It was a pivotal time for poor ol' Wallace. Because, I mean, them women in the whorehouses, most of them shipped in from Spokane, Washington—they donated to the high school, they bought band uniforms, they bought cheerleading uniforms for the school district, they bought cop cars for the local constables, and they were part of the community. This was way before anybody ever heard of AIDS, and there were no rapes or anything, so everybody was fine with it. The county sheriff was fine with it, the citizens were fine with it. But the FBI—they called them "Fun Busters Incorporated" when they come in, because everything changed then, and Wallace had to grow up. It was a tough time for the lifestyle around here.

Max: Damn, that is so fascinating. I'm thinking about how we were talking earlier about some of the folks you grew up with who are really conservative. And I think that, just in a general cultural sense, when people think of Idaho they tend to think more conservative. But the history you're telling kind of shows that there was always a richer life to the towns there—like where you are in Wallace—than we give Idaho credit for. In that history, it's not as simple as saying people there are inherently conservative and prudish. Actually, it was the FBI in '91 that kind of forced that conservative culture onto a town that didn't have it as much before.

Rick: You might be right there. As far as the political part of it, I think it was split right down the middle the whole way. Like I say, I wasn't a politically minded person until, I don't know, maybe when Obama got in there. Maybe I started listening to it a little bit then. But right now, yeah, this is a red state, and they just carry it way too far. I mean, I'm not a Trumper. My brother is, but we've learned . . . we love each other, and we get on the phone and we talk and we don't bark at each other's opinions. We get along that way. But there's a lot of guys here in this town I've had to back away from, because they just get their feelings hurt, and I'm not losing friends over the whole thing. But yeah, it's hard to say the way this town was and what the politics were. When I was brought up my dad told me, because I was asking the difference between Democrat and Republican, "Well, Republicans are the companies and the Democrats are the laborers." That's kind of how I thought things were. I guess it wasn't quite that simple.

Max: That's something that resonates with me quite a bit. Because even though I didn't realize it when I was growing up, I did learn later in life that the side of my family that was almost entirely Democrat, the Mexican side—they were almost all union workers. On the Republican side, though, no one was really a union worker, and that included our family. I never made that connection when I was growing up, but it's something I've been thinking a lot about now. Why don't we talk a little more about that? You said that you were at the Bunker Hill zinc plant in '76, then you ended up leaving on . . . not the rosiest of terms [laughs]. Then you started working as a miner in '79. I always love asking this question . . . because, honestly, I know jack shit about what it's like to work in a silver mine, or a zinc plant, or anything like that . . . What's the job like? What is it like when you're down there in the mines? And what was it like for you just getting accustomed to doing that work?

Rick: The one thing I knew when I first came over here is that miners made good money, but I didn't know anything about mining. Even just hearing about it . . . to think that I could do that myself was a little bit intimidating. But I went on a tour at the old Star mine up there. In fact, the friend that I grew up with in Clark Fork was working as an electrician in one of the mines and he took me on a tour. I crawled up these ladders up into this stope . . . that's where the vein is . . . and the first guy I seen was about five-six and 135 pounds! When I thought about miners, I guess I had the Hulk in mind or something. But when I seen this little guy I thought, "Well, Jesus, if he could do it, so could I." [Laughs]. Even before that, though, there was just a general sense of respect for miners, so you had that in the back of your head all the time too.

So I got a chance, and I went underground. Having my background and my work ethic, I knew what these guys wanted—they just wanted hard work. And I was never, ever afraid of hard work. I was playing in a couple different basketball leagues at the time and I had a traveling team that I ran around with up in Canada and Montana, so I was fit. And I worked a little bit logging in the woods too, so I knew how to high step, which is important because with mining you're always under the gun. You don't do a blast every day—it depends on what your job is—but you have to do so much work in a day's time; back then it was eight hours. The miners knew if a guy was going to be worth a crap within a day, pretty much. Usually you give a guy a week before you shit-can 'em [laughs], but you knew if a guy had potential or not pretty damn quick, and I'm not so sure that loggers don't know the same thing. And construction workers too—they probably know pretty damn fast whether a guy's gonna make it or not.

Anyway, I worked my butt off to get my job done. At the time I was basically a miner's helper. You get all their wood back there, their timber, what they call "lag." They're like big, three-inch-thick boards, rough cut, anywhere from six inches wide, maybe even ten to twelve inches wide, and they might be six feet long, twelve feet long—whatever they need up there—and you ship that up to them. And once they got all the help that they needed from you, *then* you could go up there and learn how to mine. That was my goal every day: to get my job done, make them happy, then get up there and learn how to mine, because that's where the money was. And I didn't even work very long at all as a "nipper" . . . that's the miner's helper . . . before they handed me a drill and I went to work in the stopes. Then it's just a matter of making as much money as you can per year.

That mine was pretty deep already. It was down over eight thousand feet deep. It was basically a zinc mine that had been going since the early 1900s. But zinc wasn't as high in demand as silver, so that mine pretty much shut down. They only go so deep, then it costs too much to get the rock to the surface. And so I went to another mine that really wasn't too far away, as the crow flies, but it was a silver mine. That was the Lucky Friday mine up in Mullan, which is really close to the Montana border. I spent the rest of my career up there. That was, let's see . . . forty years I mined altogether, three of them at the Star and then thirty-seven at the Lucky Friday.

Once I got over to Lucky Friday we went to shift work, different shifts of guys cycling in and out throughout the day. At the Star we was working straight days and you could live life the way it's supposed to be lived. You could work, you could go to your bowling league on Tuesday night, then go back to work hungover on Wednesday. But it was still a great mine to work at, and all of the bosses were guys who had worked their way up through the ranks. They were rank-and-file, and they had the respect of everybody. Nowadays you get these little pimple-face farts that come out of engineering school and they never really had hands-on experience.

Max: Mmhmm.

Rick: They're great at the bookwork and all that, but they come in there and it's just . . . some of them are alright, and some of them aren't, but the respect just isn't the same. And they look at labor differently too, because they haven't been there. They just look at labor as an expenditure that they have to deal with. Modern-day management is so much different than it was before. It's just hard to take it. You know, I've lived my mining life with that respect of management and labor. Not that there wasn't differences—there's always differences. But the history of unions in this valley is pretty radical too, especially in the early days. There was one mill . . . the workers just blew it up . . . because they brought in scabs during one of their labor disputes. They were pretty radical back then. [Laughs.]

Max: [Laughs.]

Rick: They actually started a firefight. There were guns going back and forth, and that was almost a distraction so the other guys could get in there, set the charges, and blow up the place. The feds come in on that one too. They had martial law and they had bullpens set up as makeshift jails down there in Wallace. They had all kinds of guys in jail over that. Shit, they even hijacked a train and a bunch of them got on it and went to Bunker Hill, which is another fifteen miles away from Wallace, and they set some dynamite charges there and blew up part of the Bunker Hill! That's the way they were back then. And the way they are now [laughs] . . . we're pretty tame these days.

Max: [Laughs.]

Rick: The problem these days is they got cameras all over the place. You ain't gonna get away with nothing these days.

Max: Right.

Rick: It's just a little different. See, my father-in-law—he was a miner too back in the day. Like I say, I was at the tail end of the rowdy days of Wallace with all the gambling and stuff, but he was right in the heart of it. When all's said and done, I'm not sure he was really all that proud of some of the things he did, but he had some stories to tell. I had to drag them out of him, but he had some stories to tell of the Wild West days of Wallace.

Max: I bet! God, there's just so much running through my mind right now. One of the other things that really struck me was how you described the ways management has changed over the years, over your own career. That's something that really resonates. I'll be honest, I've heard so many people in so many different industries describe similar things. I remember talking to a woman who's my age, about thirty-four, named Jami. She's a shipbuilder in Maine, and we talked about how she and her coworkers at Bath Iron Works went on strike, *during the pandemic*, for most of the summer. And one of the things that the workers there talked about was how these new managers who were being hired were academically smart, book smart, but they had never worked in the shipyard. They didn't respect all the years of accrued knowledge that the old timers had and would need to pass on to the newer, younger folks in the union. That just wasn't as much of a concern for the new managers. And I've even heard the same thing from doctors and nurses at hospitals who say, "We're working in this new 'retail health' model, where you have this top-down bureaucracy of well-educated managers who are telling physicians what to do and how long it should take, even though they've never been in an operating room themselves." And it's just . . . you start to see this weird thing pouring over the country like water—this weird management ideology that doesn't have any kind of sense of what it means to be a worker or what impact your decisions are going to have on people's lives and bodies.

Rick: Yeah. That's exactly the way you lose that essential respect too. I remember one guy, he was a mining engineer and they knew they were grooming him to move up through the ranks. He put himself down as a nipper for me and my partner, because we were mining and he wanted to be our helper. And he nipped for us for months because he wanted to get hands-on. He earned a lot of respect for doing that, and that place runs so much better with a guy like that.

See, the history of this place, like I just told you, was pretty radical at times when they had union disputes. But from the time that I started, like early '80s, there really wasn't that many disputes that weren't settled before the contract was up. And one of those disputes took place at my father-in-law's house. He wasn't even an officer of the union, but he was kind of one of the main guys up there at the mine. The mine manager went to my father-in-law's house and they went down in his den. He had a beautiful den there. He was a hunter and he had mounts all over the place. One of the most beautiful dens I've ever seen in my life. He had a couple grand slam sheep up there on the walls, mule deer and white-tailed deer and upland game—just beautiful. They all sat down there, got a bottle of whiskey, and they settled the labor dispute right there. That's how they did it. There was nothing official about it. And that's how they settled those disputes, because that's how much respect they had for each other.

Now, I just came off of a two-and-a-half-year strike. It's actually the longest strike that we've ever had in the history of this valley, and it was ugly. There was a loss of respect there that I'm not sure they could ever get back. The reason the mine went on strike originally was because they wanted to "modernize" the mine. They wanted to be at the "forefront of technology." Well, this is all a big narrative that they wanted their investors to listen to, but it was just a bullshit story—nothing's ever going to happen there. This mine, the Lucky Friday mine that Hecla [Mining Company] has up there right now in Mullan, is a little over nine thousand feet deep.

Max: Wow.

Rick: At some point the problem is Mother Nature has a vein down there that's getting wider and higher silver content as it goes down, which is great, but to mine it at that depth takes a lot of investment. So, it's a hell of a time to be changing the technique of mining. Mining is about change, so it's not like we're scared to change or anything, but what they're trying to do is bring in new equipment when you're really in the eleventh hour of a mine's life. It just didn't make a lot of sense.

Anyway, they've changed their reasoning for having that labor dispute three or four different times, and they still haven't got the equipment they said they were going to get here. Shit, I don't know, it was supposed to show up a couple years ago and it still isn't here, last I heard. They put it off for another year. They wanted wide, sweeping cuts and everything, because they were gonna have this new technology come in and they needed that extra money. The thing is, we didn't ask for anything in our new contract. We just wanted a continuation of our own old contract, which hadn't been changed for six years. We just wanted another six years of that. Because they did invest in a new shaft to go deeper on that vein and that cost a lot of money. They put $250 million into that new shaft. And when they do that they provide jobs, and we appreciate that, so we didn't ask for anything. It's not like the unions have to be against the company all the time, you know? We were willing to work with them, not ask for anything, and just go back to work. But that wasn't good enough for them. They want to make cuts to our benefits, make cuts to our wages, and it just wasn't gonna fly. So we went on a two-and-a-half-year strike and basically ended up having to give in to them. Not totally—they had to give up some stuff too. But they started bringing in scabs, and there were a few of our guys who crossed the picket line also, so it kind of fell apart after all that time. We had a vote and it narrowly passed.

So we went back to work, and I just went back for five months—just long enough to be a needle in their ass. I had planned on retiring during that strike, and I would have retired anyways, but I just went back for a little while to . . . I don't know, maybe to prove something to myself. I'm not sure. But it was just ugly the way it went down. There were a lot of issues during that strike. A couple of our guys got fired for things that they did. There were some confrontations. The only reason there wasn't more things that happened is, like I told you before, they brought in a camera crew and set up cameras all over the place, which was one of the smartest things they did. There wasn't any sneaking around.

Max: Yeah, I guess they read their history about mines getting blown up in the past . . .

Rick: Oh, yeah. That was one of our calls: "Remember the Frisco!" Because that was the old Frisco mill that got blown to smithereens back in the day. So "Remember the Frisco!" was one of the posters that we had.

Max: That's pretty badass, though.

Rick: But, like I say, this was one of those disputes that could have been settled pretty damn quickly if they would have sat down with a little damn respect to work the damn thing out. But the CEO of this company—he's not a miner. He was a lawyer and an accountant. He could give a damn about this mine's product. We could be making tennis shoes up there and he would run the place the same way. It's just a business to him. He doesn't have that mining background. He's the first CEO that didn't have that mining background and, boy, you can tell it. Well, actually, he *did* have a mining background—I think he was the CFO of another mine in Montana. And to this day they have cyanide and some other chemical leaking out of the ground up there that the Montana taxpayers have to take care of, because the mine went bankrupt and they only put so much aside for reclamation. When something like that happens, after whatever they set aside is done and they go bankrupt, they're not even an entity anymore. The taxpayers have to pick up the tab. This CEO—he just goes to another company, makes his millions, and I guarantee you he hasn't lost one ounce of sleep over all that goddamn environmental destruction he left behind in Montana. I sound a little bit like a disgruntled worker . . . and that's because I am.

Max: Well, shit, man, I think you got every right to be!

Rich: Well, I do. I tell you, I was all over the country throughout this strike. I was one of the guys who didn't work. A lot of our guys went out and got other jobs, because miners are in high demand, especially, like, a mining mechanic. A good mining mechanic can make a lot of money just about anywhere, and experienced miners are in demand. So there was no lack of mining jobs, but I was one of the guys who stayed back and just fought the fight. I was all over, hearing about different labor disputes from folks in the U.S. and Canada. And they all have the same problems! Maybe different particulars, but basically the same problems with management and labor: lack of trust and respect. It really isn't that hard to settle them damn things if you have that respect. But to sit there and shut down a mine, to idle a mine for over two years, is just ignorant, absolutely ignorant. I mean, they kept going a little bit with the salaried people that they had up there, but it's lucky somebody didn't get hurt real bad by doing that. But the thing is, once a mine shuts down everything gets rusty, all the pipes and everything. You got to keep everything pumped out, you got to keep air flowing. There's a lot to shutting something down, and to starting it back up.

Max: Man, and you know what's kind of blowing my mind about all of this? We haven't even talked about the COVID-19 pandemic, but that's really the epilogue to this two-year strike, right? You said you went back for five months after the strike ended, but you finally retired in August . . .

Rick: Yeah, as soon as the strike got over . . . that's basically when COVID cranked up. And they consider mining an "essential industry," so it wasn't going to affect the mine as far as shutting it down. But they did have to try different things. If you went in a door, for example, you couldn't come out of that door. The precautions that they took weren't really adhered to. We would wear a mask on the surface, but as soon as we got underground . . . I mean, it's hotter than hell down there in some places, too hot to put a mask over your face. And a lot of the time you're kind of by yourself anyway. There might be another guy a few hundred feet away. It really doesn't make a lot of sense to keep a mask on down there. As far as COVID affecting the day-to-day activity in the mine, it's fairly minimal, and they're pretty lax about it.

Max: Mmhmm.

Rick: Now, I haven't been up there since August, so maybe that's changed a little bit. But I know the Panhandle Health District down here is kind of calling the shots on it, so if they ever got to the point where the Health District wasn't happy with what they were doing up at the mine they could shut them down. Whatever the Panhandle Health District wants from the mine the mine will do to stay open. Basically, the main thing is everybody gets their temperature checked. Every day, when you pull into the parking lot, they put a little gun up to your head and check your temperature and ask if you want a mask. That's kind of it, really. You wear a mask while you're on the surface, but as soon as you get underground you just pretty much take it off and go to work. So, it really didn't have a big impact—easy to get around, anyway.

Max: Yeah. If you think about it, if the highest risk places are crowded spaces with low ventilation, then if you're working on your own in a mine and you're quite a ways away from somebody else, I guess that's one of the safer places you could be. Maybe "safe" isn't the right word, but . . .

Rick: And also, there's always ventilation in a mine. Well, in most places there's ventilation. The entrance to the mine has air going down, then at some point, depending on how big the mine is, there's some intermediate fans that are pulling that air through the mine, through all the workplaces, and then it has an outlet going out through another shaft. You have air moving all the time that way—it's not like it's stagnant in there or you're breathing each other's air.

Max: Has it been much different outside of the mine? I can only imagine where your head was at a year ago when you're just coming off this two-year strike, which didn't go the way you wanted, you were already thinking of retiring . . . and then this pandemic hits. Could you try to go back to that point and talk about what it was like for you and your wife as the reality of COVID-19 was setting in?

Rick: For myself, I guess you'd call what I'm doing "quarantining," but this is kind of my lifestyle anyway. I live out here in the country and I'm just, you know, learning how to play guitar. I'm just happy being right here— until my fishing season starts, then I'll start doing that. In fact, I'm looking for a German Shorthaired right now so I can get back into pheasant hunting. I lost my dog here a few years back and I haven't got another one. I think I got one more dog in me. So, I'm basically cooped up here voluntarily this time of year.

Now my wife—she's going all the time. She's kind of a caregiver for her mother, who has medical issues, and her sister also has medical issues. She's running around and in contact with other people all the time, but she always wears a mask. She's pretty careful that way. But it would be her to bring something back if we were going to get it. But I just . . . personally, I don't have any fear of it whatsoever. And I do have lung problems too. If I was to catch it I would probably have an issue, because I have silicosis from the mines. They suspected that I had it for a few years—since 2012, actually—but I just didn't have it diagnosed. Once I had it diagnosed that was it, I just stopped mining.

Around here people I know have been testing positive, but they're usually younger guys and they don't even have symptoms. I think we've been pretty lucky around here—anyone that I know, anyway. In Coeur d'Alene—I forget the population, but it's over fifty thousand—they've been getting a lot of cases. But this is a small town, a lot of us are rural, and I just don't hear anybody really worrying about it much.

Max: Well, you know, when you've got a community that is very attached to the mining industry, and a lot of families with folks who work in the mines, I guess silicosis is a much bigger threat to that community than COVID-19 is right now?

Rick: I'll tell you what, I know a lot of guys have retired from that mine and didn't last long after that. But I don't think a lot of them ever had it diagnosed. They just had breathing problems, went and got oxygen, and never held the mine accountable for it. I don't think this mine has ever been held accountable. Now, my claim is going through the state right now, because I wrote it up as an industrial illness, and I don't know how it's gonna turn out. I haven't heard back yet, but I got a feeling I'll probably end up with a lawyer and going through all that. But you're right. A lot of people, I'm sure, have died because of it. But COVID itself? I don't know. I don't think that's going to be too much of an issue around here.

9. Ashley Powell

My name is Ashley Powell. I am thirty-two years old. I was born in Houston, Texas, and then my family moved to Pennsylvania, back where they are from. I was, till eighteen, raised outside Pittsburgh, then I had a falling out with my parents, became the black sheep of my family, and moved to Florida for seven years. Then I had a quarter-life crisis, hated everything in Florida, and randomly moved to Portland, Oregon.

Max: Now, I'm no stranger to the quarter-life crisis [laughs]. I'm always curious to hear other people's experiences with it . . .

Ashley: Oh, yeah, I just got rid of everything and moved out here. It's funny because once you're away from things you get nostalgic for them. I miss the beach so much, for example, and I even kind of miss the trashiness of the people at times, you know?

Max: Oh, definitely. I feel the same way about Southern California, which is where I grew up. No matter where I go in the world, no matter how long I've been gone, I always miss the beach. I know it's cliché, but there is something almost primordial about that feeling in your gut, in your soul, when you hear the waves crashing and feel the sun on your face—it just feels like home. I really do miss it. To your point, though, there are even times when I start to miss the things that I always hated about Southern California, like the sort of power-washed stucco and synthetic sheen that makes all the strip malls and promenades look the same. I find myself getting homesick for it.

Ashley: I should also preface that I lived in Pensacola, which is up in the panhandle. They actually call that "L.A.," which stands for "Lower

Alabama," so it's a little different than the rest of Florida. It's got, like, slightly more rednecky vibes. It's interesting, though, because Pensacola is not a huge tourist destination, the beaches aren't partied on and they're totally pristine and beautiful!

Max: So, why Florida? Was there anything specific that brought you down there, or did you just throw a dart at a map? [Laughs.]

Ashley: I had some friends down there and a guy I had a thing for (it obviously didn't work). I had gotten a job at Lowe's as a cashier, then they switched me to an office job. Minimum wage was $7.75 but they hired me on at $12.50, so I thought I was making great money as an eighteen-year-old with no experience. I had also gotten into a lot of struggles with my mom. She has some mental illness issues, to put it lightly. A big reason why I moved is I was arguing with my parents. They wouldn't fill out the FAFSA [Free Application for Federal Student Aid] for me because my mother hadn't filed her taxes in years, and I was having problems talking to the local college about how I could declare myself an independent. So I just kind of gave up on college for a while. After that I worked at Lowe's for years, I did some waitressing jobs, then I got a job for a local moving company that was actually a franchise. I worked there for five years. I was really good at that job. I had a lot of friends and we would hang out a lot at the beach and bars, and I was living a pretty good life till I just woke up one day and was like, "No, I can't do this anymore."

Max: Do you know what made you feel that way?

Ashley: Like I was saying before, I lived in Pennsylvania for eight years, Texas for seven years, and Florida for seven years, but I view Florida as my home, because that's where I fully formed as an adult, learned how to pay bills, and became an actualized person. That being said—and this sounds cliché to say—I feel like nothing for me will ever feel like home. I honestly think I have two more years of Portland left in me and then I've gotta bounce. I guess this is why I want to get a job in tech. I never want to be married to a place, because things just start to feel stale. I might move back down to Texas . . . Arizona doesn't sound that bad. I don't know. There's just a lot of places I want to live, and nowhere will ever feel like the right place.

Max: I think that's probably more of a common experience for people in our generation than we realize. I don't necessarily know why that is, though . . .

Ashley: I'm sure it's got something to do with having fucked-up parents that you feel never loved you or something like that.

Max: Yeah, that might be a part of it [laughs].

Ashley: [Laughs.] I feel like that's what my therapist would probably say to me. "Yeah, your parents didn't love you, so that's probably why you gotta keep moving and looking for love." But, I mean, it's more than that. Because I've genuinely loved every place I've ever been, but but I just . . . maybe it's also commitment issues. And that's definitely a thing for our generation for sure: Is the grass always greener on that other side? I feel like there's a lot of that.

Max: I think you're right. And like you said, it's probably a mix of things. Obviously our own personal upbringings play into it, but we also grew up in an era when, from kindergarten on up, the future was sold to us in a very particular way. We were always taught to focus on the *next steps*, I guess, and we were never taught to appreciate where we were. We've always been working *toward* something—working through elementary school to get to junior high, working through junior high to get to high school, working through high school to get to college or to get a job. Then you've got to focus on moving from this position at work to another one, or from this job to a better one, or from this position in society to the one above it. There's just no real sense of being home in our lives. We weren't really raised to feel grounded where we are, ever.

Ashley: I feel there's a part of me that's like, "Well, I didn't go to college, so I'll never be complete." But there's also a part of me that's like, "Holy shit, I'm not in college debt! I have no debts." And I'm somebody who would probably be totally fine not having kids. If you ever met me in person, I'm not somebody who you would think would ever have a kid. But I feel like I would not be complete unless I do those things. Like, I *want* a kid, but I want a dude to stay home and raise it so I don't have to [laughs]. I want one, but I only want it because I feel like that was what was sold to me: "*That's* how you go be happy."

Max: What you just said really clicked with me, because now I'm also wondering how this all connects to the economic situation of our generation. We grew up hearing all these stories about what makes a good life, what makes a happy and successful life, right? But the older I got the fewer opportunities there actually were for us to build that good life. From the social safety net that used to exist to the steady jobs that you could support a family on, previous generations had more opportunities for getting that economic security, more opportunities to build that good life. And they weren't buried in debt. We don't have that. And so, it's kind of like we're all trying to grasp at pieces and shards of that dream. Like you said, it could be kids, it could be living in a certain place, it could be traveling, it could be having a certain job—but at the end of the day we're basically trying to cobble together a collage of that good life without ever really having the economic ability to sustain it.

Ashley: Yeah. I definitely grew up with my parents not coming to a lot of my softball games or cross country meets, because my dad worked out of town and he always sucked up any overtime he could get. Also I have three brothers and they were involved in a bunch of activities too. But the thing is, with his position, he worked for the same company for thirty years. That's something that we don't have anymore. That's not a thing!

Max: No, absolutely not.

Ashley: It is not a thing at all right now. He has a pension! He pretty much had to retire early because of COVID, because he was scared of losing part of his pension. But he's fine. His house is paid for, he just got himself a dog, and he's just chillin'. He's only fifty-six. He's bored.

Max: And that's the thing, right? That used to be way more commonplace. It used to be a reasonable expectation that we could all live with that level of comfort. Not anymore. Even the very notion of a pension is so alien to so many of us.

Ashley: Exactly. And I've read articles about people moving from job to job. You work a year somewhere, you get your experience there, then you go see what this other job has to offer. You even see that in the service and hospitality industry. There's definitely a hierarchy when it comes to bartenders, and you do see people moving around and trying to climb their way up the ladder.

Max: Let's talk about that—let's connect those two ends of the story and get to your work as a bartender. So, you woke up in Florida one day and you just knew that your time there was done and that it was time to move on. Then what happened?

Ashley: I found a job with a moving company out here, because I didn't want to move somewhere without having a job. It was very low paying, and once I got out here I found out they had lied to me about how much money I would be making on commission. It wasn't a very well-run franchise. But in my first month here I got a job at a local bar. It's a dive bar where you get a lot of regulars, and it's a karaoke bar. They also show a lot of sports and UFC matches. It's been around for like thirty years. It's a great place. But I didn't know all of that when I started working there. I just got the job there and started out part-time, then I realized, "Holy shit, I make way more money serving and bartending than I do at this dumb moving company and I don't want to do this anymore." So I stopped doing that and went full-time bartending. And I love it. It's great. I feel like I am a stereotype of a bartender in a way: I'm five-three, 125 pounds, I'm scarier than any bouncer you'll ever meet. I'm very boisterous, I have a lot of opinions and I joke around a lot. I'm also going to sit and have a drink with you when I'm done with my shift. I could be in any movie, any sitcom, and be *that* person, you know what I mean?

Max: [Laughs.] Yup.

Ashley: Like, I'm very well aware of what I am [laughs]. Honestly, I think being a bartender is the easiest job when it's easy and the hardest job when it's not. I work at a bar that's slightly on the outskirts of the city. And I don't know if you've heard about it, but there's a homeless problem in Portland, and that problem has a lot to do with people not getting the proper pathways and help for their mental illness. So, I've had people take swings at me, people who just come in the bar and scream or tell me they're gonna punch me in my face—all kinds of crazy shit. But yeah, my job's easy when it's easy and it's hard when it's hard, but I love it. And I've worked part-time at other bars in town too. I can definitely make you any classic cocktail you want, and I can also pour you ten vodka sodas real fast. That's kind of where I am with everything. And I'm very lucky, too, that my boss provides health insurance. In the hospitality industry, unless you work for a corporate chain, that's not a thing.

Max: No, it really isn't! I sure as hell didn't get health care when I was serving [laughs]. I'm kind of blown away by that.

Ashley: Yeah, my boss—he's fucking great. He's part Canadian and part Korean, so I guess we're technically a minority-owned business. But yeah, he's great, and I'm just very lucky to have my job.

Max: I wanted to pick up on something you said, because I think the way you put it makes a ton of sense. I've never been a bartender, but I've been a server, I've been a delivery driver, I've worked at a frozen yogurt place and a Mexican spot called Pepe's. And what you said is spot on. When it's easy it's the easiest job in the world, but the hard parts can be very, very hard. And that's just me speaking from my own experience. I've also heard so many stories from other friends and coworkers in the service industry about all the harassment, even assault, and other bullshit people face. So not only are you dealing with that day-to-day crapshoot of customers being nice or being dicks, but for someone like you—like you said, you're a petite woman working at a bar—there's probably a lot of additional crap that you have to wade through on a daily basis.

Ashley: Yeah, but it's still fun. Something different every day.

Max: Yeah, that's true. And maybe that's one of the real draws of working at a dive bar, right? Like you said, you get to have an actual relationship and build a rapport with the regulars who come in. You don't get to really have any meaningful relationships with people like that in many other types of work. I admit, I kind of miss that.

Ashley: Yeah. I will say, though, being that it's a karaoke bar . . . I used to work weekend nights, and that's a completely different animal compared to the happy-hour professionals who are coming in for a snack and, like, two drinks with their coworkers. I always say it's a bar where you don't just have one or two drinks—you have a few. And I've seen people *drunk*. But now, since I've worked there five years, I work more happy hour shifts. It was kind of a joke for a while, like, "Oh, Ashley, you don't have to work those karaoke nights anymore!" I can pick and choose my shifts more because I'm old now. I'm thirty-two. I'm an old bartender [laughs].

Max: [Laughs.]

Ashley: I'm lucky to have that seniority at my position, and I don't have to deal with the weekend drama. And, you know, enough chaos happens during the day too . . .

Max: I was gonna ask you about that everyday chaos. I'm assuming many people reading this have never worked as a bartender and don't really know all the things your job entails. Before the COVID-19 pandemic, what did a typical week or day look like for you?

Ashley: I normally work Sunday through Wednesday, and back then it used to be worked out with our boss that we would work really long shifts for four days so that we could have three days off—and everyone loved it. I probably talk more than any of my coworkers, and people come in because they want to talk, not counting the karaoke nights. They want to sit at the bar and they want to talk. That's one thing I have noticed after COVID. Girls don't normally go out to bars by themselves. There are a few types of girls that do, like me—I'm one of them. But men will go to a bar by themselves all the time just to have an interaction, whether they're single men or men who are in relationships. You know, they don't have to worry about being raped and murdered primarily. But when we did reopen the bar I noticed that all of my single clientele dudes were not coming in. They don't feel comfortable coming in anymore because they can't sit at the bar.

One of the reasons I love this job, as I've loved previous jobs in the past, is my boss trusts us and there is no micromanagement. It's definitely a bar where you do everything. You are essentially the bartender who runs all the food, handles all the money, makes all of the drinks. We also have lotto machines—do you have those in Baltimore?

Max: We do not, but I remember seeing them in Portland.

Ashley: They are a blessing and a curse evenly. You'll see a homeless guy outside begging for money, then an hour later you'll see him inside putting it in the machines just hoping to break even, and you might find a needle on the ground after you go back there and check. It's a mess. We also had a customer urinate on himself once while he was playing a machine. It definitely attracts a clientele that is not as savory, I guess one would say? On the other hand, it also attracts people who are very generous, because when they win they view it as, like, luck? Free money? I'm not sure. Gambling has never been a real thing for me. But the most I've ever gotten tipped in a day—I think I made $500 once off somebody just from their lotto winnings. But hey, that's rare. That's not an all-the-time thing. I'm not balling by any means. And you don't see a lot of machines in cocktail bars here—they're always in dive bars. Honestly, Max, it's hard for me to remember what the previous times were like now that I'm thinking of it . . .

Max: I think it feels that way for a lot of us, really. We've been going through this for a year now, and life before that feels so long ago . . . it's hard to even put ourselves back in that position and remember who we were. You were talking about how you would whip up a bunch of drinks really quickly, handle money, take a lot of different drink orders from different people coming into the bar, etc. So, are you what they call a mixologist?

Ashley: No, I would not call myself a mixologist. I am a badass bartender! But we can talk about your flavor profiles, we can talk about your favorite shot, your favorite type of liquors, and I'm sure I can make you anything you want. I learned so much from other bartenders I've worked with. I've been very, very lucky because I've worked with all different types, and I've worked with people who probably consider themselves mixologists. I feel like true bartenders hate that term, though—do you know that?

Max: Well, I *do* know that the one guy who proudly called himself a mixologist at the restaurant I worked at in Chicago was a real douchebag [laughs].

Ashley: Yeah [laughs], there we go. So, yeah, we're not a mixologist place, we're a bar. When my boss was iinterviewing me for the job he said it's kind of like a *Cheers* bar place, and I was like, "Okay, I've never seen *Cheers*, whatever." And then I started working there, and I was actually really timid and shy at first, because all these people knew each other and I was the new person. I'm the complete opposite now, and everyone here is very friendly. There used to be this thing where a lot of Portland bars were known for their "Portland service," which is essentially when the bartender acts annoyed that you asked for a drink and that they have to get off their phone and help you, and they still expect a 20 percent or more tip. The bar I work at, you don't get that service. Everyone I work with is super nice. We're happy to help you—that's our job.

I'm more of a gregarious, fun bartender. People are coming to me to have a good time. They're not coming to me because I make this or that really good drink. I mean, I *can*, and I have had customers compliment me on my beverages. But if you want to spend fifteen bucks on a cocktail you know where you're supposed to be. Our bar is a read-your-environment kind of place. It's not a place where we have a wine list, though I have been asked. I've had people ask for the wine list and I'm just like, "No" [laughs].

Max: [Laughs.] I'll take a dive bar over an expensive cocktail bar any day. Well, let's move from "the before times" to this endless, anxious hell we've been stewing in for the past year. I know it's hard to recall what we were doing and how we were processing everything as the reality of the COVID-19 pandemic really took over, but do you remember what it was like for you? In your corner of the world, living in Portland, working as a bartender, what was your experience of all this?

Ashley: It *has* been almost a year, huh? I remember . . . I think it was the end of December or the beginning of January . . . people were posting on Reddit about this weird virus in China. And I was like, "Well, that's weird. No one's been talking about this over here." Because, I mean, working at a bar, people talk about current situations. So I did some more reading on it and I saw what the Chinese government was doing with their lockdowns, and I was like, "Holy shit, this is about to come here." I'm already known for being really cautious with germs and handling cash, because we all know how dirty cash is, and we deal with a lot of cash from those lotto machines, but I was just more aware of it than ever and really on edge about it.

I remember going into work and telling all of my coworkers, "Hey, just so you know, there's this virus in China and it's pretty much here now—it's in Seattle and California. We're about to be laid off. Everything's gonna shut down." And they were like, "No. No way." And I also remember watching this woman . . . goddamn it if her name isn't Karen [laughs] . . . Karen was sitting at the bar talking to another boy, and they both had a few drinks, and she ended up sharing her food with him while we were talking about COVID. I was like, "Oh, yeah, we're about to shut down." And she's like, "Well, I think you're an idiot." And I was just like, "Okay, lady." [Laughs.]

Max: [Laughs.] Wow.

Ashley: "Okay, *Karen*. Here's your wine." I didn't say anything mean back, because it was just so funny to me. I've been called "fat bitch," "dumb cunt," and "stupid whore" so many times that "idiot" is nothing. "Thank you, Karen."

Eventually my coworkers started taking it more and more seriously, and next thing you know our governor, Kate Brown, shut everything down on March 16 for the first lockdown. And she got a lot of shit for it from the hospitality industry. March 16 is the day right before St. Patrick's Day. I see where she was coming from, trying to stop a lot of what would be huge gatherings. However, you have all of these businesses that have all of this product, all of this unprepared food, which all costs money, not knowing what to do because she said, "No, you have to shut down tomorrow." And my boss was one of those generous people. He was just like, "Okay, well, come get all the food. Take it home." So we're back there in the kitchen dividing up portions. Because what is he going to do? Just let all that food stay there and rot? But that's money that all these business owners just had to watch disappear, which is terrible. And then Kate Brown, bless her heart—she did this thing where she would open and then close, then tease re-opening, and then it was like, "You can only stay open till ten o'clock. No, stay open till eleven o'clock. Only outdoor dining, though." The only way I can explain it, I guess, is that it felt like being a dog on a leash that just wants to be told which way to go. Like, we'll do whatever you want, but you're just being cruel and pulling the leash the other way every time we try to follow you. Some of her decisions didn't make sense. And then you have your friends lighting people up on social media while all this was going on like, "If you don't believe in COVID, if you don't wear a mask, UNFRIEND ME NOW." Remember when Trump was elected? "If you believe in Trump, UNFRIEND ME NOW." There was a lot of that same weird signaling going on.

Max: I remember seeing some of that.

Ashley: Yeah, it was weird. When the lockdown started to happen I stopped spending money on anything I didn't need, because I was like, "Oh, this is really happening." But also because I'm, like, a very paranoid person, and I guess that finally worked out for me this one time. I'm normally really financially irresponsible. I have no idea why that is. But I had actually saved up some money. I had talked about taking a trip to New Zealand, I was looking at coding bootcamps, so I had a little bit of money saved up.

You said you've worked jobs in the hospitality industry too, so you know that most of these people live paycheck to paycheck. They party as hard as they work, but these people don't have any kind of backup or savings. And then you have the problem with Oregon unemployment. I guess the state had gotten millions of dollars ten years ago from the government to fix their unemployment system, and they never did. I had friends who had no money, they couldn't pay their bills, and there was no help. I had friends putting auto-dialers on their phone trying to get through to the unemployment office. *Eventually* the unemployment payments went through, but for me and most of my friends it was five weeks later. Five weeks later! I was also in a lucky position at that time because I lived with roommates. Like I said, I was trying to save money, and they're also my really good friends—I treasure them so much. I lived in a house that they owned, so my rent was dirt cheap.

There was also this feeling in the air during the first lockdown that was like, "Oh, shit, we're all gonna die. This is the virus that kills all of us." There was a lot of fearmongering in the news too. And, I mean, I don't blame the media for that at the time, because no one really knew what was going on in the beginning, back in March. No one knew. I understand erring on the side of caution, but I definitely thought we were all gonna die. I'm really healthy, I work out, and I take my vitamins, so I wasn't so much worried for myself. But when I'm bartending I deal with people's beverages and food . . . what if I got it and I gave it to somebody? What if they died? Or had residual damage? That's a horrible feeling to have. I assumed I'd be one of the people who got it. I was just thinking, "I'm going to get it. I'm going to be one of the first people to get it, because I talk to so many people every week." But with the "we're all gonna die" stuff happening I was like, "Okay, I'm going to go stay with my boyfriend." I had just rekindled things with an ex-boyfriend back in January and things were going really well, so I ended up going to stay with him, but all of my friends were on lockdown. There really was a sense that this was like the apocalypse though. That's what it felt like. You remember that, right? The toilet paper was gone?!

Max: Yeah! And you couldn't get hand sanitizer for weeks.

Ashley: Yeah, it was one of those things you'd make kind of fucked-up jokes to your friends about, like, "Is this a good time to get into the funeral business?" And my boyfriend and I—we would go grocery shopping once a week and try to buy extra things, you know? Just in case you literally can't leave your house at some point, or the supply chains for all these grocery stores go down.

Max: That connects to what you were saying about the unemployment office, right? My folks also had to wait weeks to get a response from unemployment, and I heard so many similar stories from friends all over the country. I know that it's kind of cliché to say at this point, now that we've been living under these conditions for so long, but I really think it's important to recognize that what this pandemic has done is lay bare for everyone just how rotted out and termite-riddled our system is. For decades these fucking politicians and powerful people have been stripping down the social safety net and giving up more and more basic government functions to "the market," and that left our whole system so unprepared and ill-equipped to handle any sort of emergency like this. This didn't just happen overnight—they've been chipping away at this shit for years, and when people needed support the most the system buckled. There was nowhere to turn—it really felt like we were all on our own. And then, like you said, you add this kind of apocalyptic feeling you got every time you would go to Target or the supermarket and you would see, like, the medicine aisles completely cleaned out, the toilet paper aisles cleaned out, all the milk in the dairy aisle gone. I remember being in a store this time last year and thinking, "Man, all our textbooks in school always showed those gray photos of breadlines and food shortages in socialist countries . . . This looks a lot like that, right?" [Laughs.]

Ashley: [Laughs.] Right! It was like, "Oh, I heard about this. Looks like it could happen here after all." That makes me think about when I was younger—I so, so wanted aliens to be real, and there's still a part of me that's like, "Well, maybe . . ."

Max: [Laughs.] I'm with you. My dad and I watch alien shows all the time.

Ashley: Nice. I bring that up because I openly joke about that stuff with my friends. Anytime there's something in the news I'm like, "I told you guys! It's been happening." I'm not a conspiracy theorist or anything, and I hate that term, but I just think about it like, "Has the government done bad things to its people in the past? Yes. Why would they not do it again?" When this first happened, for example, my thought was, "Oh, they're using this to get rid of cash," because they were definitely talking about how dirty cash was and everyone was really encouraged to use a card. I was like, "Oh, they're trying to track everything through people's cards. Great. Here we go . . ." And there was something really weird going on, especially in the beginning when everyone was just avoiding each other, you know? Like they were scared of each other. "Oh, you could have it! Stay away from me! Wear a mask and the government's gonna give you money—just stay home, stay away from your friends." With all that going on, there was definitely a part of me that was thinking about those conspiracies like, "Well, this is it. This is the thing I read about in those books when I was thirteen."

I'm glad I'm not a business owner, because if I was I would have stayed open. I think it is preposterous—and this is a very unpopular opinion to have in Portland—that your government can tell you, "No, you have to shut down, you are not allowed to make money, and we're not going to help you." That is insane to me. We had this one bar stay open in Washington. They defied the government, obviously they got a huge fine, but also a bunch of Trump supporters went out there to support them. And, I mean, if I had left my bar open I don't want a bunch of Trump supporters showing up—I don't need that kind of press, you know? Anyway, I feel like this is beating a dead horse, but the way this whole thing has become politicized is . . . insanity. I hate that I'm using the word "insane" so much, but you just look around and it's like you are in a weird *Matrix* system a lot of the time.

Max: It does feel that way, right? I found myself thinking about that at some point too. And I think it says a lot about the kind of culture we were brought up in that when I've tried to describe to people what I'm going through or what this past year has felt like I end up using movies as my main reference point. It's like, "Man, what does it mean that the best way I can describe my reality is by using fictional movies that I grew up watching?" I dunno, I haven't thought it through, but it definitely says something about the weird spectacle of American life that the things we see in movies are realer to us than whatever the hell we've been living through this past year.

Ashley: Right? And it also makes me think, like . . . you know about China's social credit system? That's another thing that makes me very nervous and scared about our future, especially with Biden coming in. They're going to put in more surveillance to keep everyone "safe." And you know how China's whole thing is, "Well, if you're not doing anything wrong, what's the matter?" I worry that's what we're doing here. After the Capitol riots, I feel like maybe this whole thing is somehow gonna turn into the Patriot Act 2.0. Is this where we give up more of our rights because, "Hey, they're just trying to keep us safe"? So, I don't . . . I don't fully trust the government. I live like three blocks from the courthouse—I actually moved downtown a couple months ago—so I was living here when all those riots were happening in the summer, and I supported them. I one-hundred-percent support Black Lives Matter. There's a part of me, though, that still doesn't understand why there weren't riots over people going five months without assistance during a pandemic. There's still a part of me that's like, "Why aren't we all at the Capitol and the White House? Where the fuck is our $2,000 stimulus check? Where the fuck is Medicare for All? Why are we the only first-world country that is having this issue?"

Max: Honestly, I wish more people were as fired up as you are about those very same questions. We *should* be fucking pissed about this shit and we *should* be in the streets. I think that's a completely reasonable response to living in the wealthiest country on Earth and getting treated with such disregard and disrespect.

You said something a minute ago that really caught my ear. I've been talking to a lot of different folks for this book, really doing my best to make sense of the past year and to understand what other people are going through and how *they're* making sense of all this. And I think that, on the surface of it, like you were saying, it's impossible to make sense out of a situation that is so senseless. What's the point of trying to find any logic here when clearly there is none? But the thing that you said that really struck me is: Whatever conclusions we come to about why this is all unfolding the way it has and where it could be going, the most glaringly obvious problem here is not that we went into lockdown to try to protect public health. . . that certainly makes sense . . . but it's the fact that millions—*tens* of millions—of people en masse were basically just told, "Okay, you're on your own. Good luck." Eventually there were some lifelines. Unemployment finally started to work, there were some extended unemployment benefits, we got one fucking stimulus check, the "eviction moratorium" was more of a stay of execution than anything, etc. But the fact of the matter is so many people lost their jobs, and their health care, and the social safety net had been rotted out for so many years that it wasn't really there to catch people when they needed it the most. And we also live in a society where the kind of public services that would have really helped people in this time of need have either been criminally underfunded or privatized. And so, if people aren't working and they're getting very little assistance from the government, especially in the early days, then they're not going to be able to get the health care they need, or the psychological or financial relief they need, or any number of things. It's because of these massive failures by the government and the market to muster any kind of humane response to this crisis that I can't blame anyone for thinking that this whole thing is one big conspiracy. Because the other explanation is that neither the government nor the market give a shit if we live or die—and that's a really painful truth to confront. If working people around the country are being told to sacrifice and they're losing their jobs, and they're still being asked to pay rent and pay bills, and we can't even guarantee people will have the basic necessities to survive, of course your mind's gonna race and you're gonna start looking for answers where you can find them. You're gonna start asking, "What is the point of all this? If this is as bad as they say but they're not giving us the kind of help that a crisis of this magnitude calls for, then is there something else going on?"

Ashley: For me, I think a large part of it has to do with the fact that I have been at home and, for the past two weeks especially, I've really been conscientiously limiting my news sources. Well, not my news sources, but the time I spend on news. But it just got to the point where I was watching the news like, "Hey, does anybody else see this huge class gap? All these senators and congresspeople—they're all millionaires, they don't give a fuck about me or my friends." It's almost gotten to a point where I'm just like, "Do I need to get into politics? Do I need to start a podcast where I start bitching about politics all the time? Do I have to do . . . something?" I don't know shit, but I know that something is wrong. That's how I feel.

One of the reasons Trump got elected was because he said the mainstream media lied to us—that's one thing he wasn't wrong about, and people liked that he called it out. The mainstream media does lie to us. I'm just so sick of it. And I'm sick of these politicians lying to us. They're just so out of touch with normal people. So out of touch. It's crazy. You see Nancy Pelosi on the screen and you're just like, "Yo, Nancy, how many poor people do you know? Nancy, how many people do you know making under thirty grand a year? Nancy, how many people do you know living under the poverty line? Nancy, how many people do you know with six kids?"

Max: For real! Out of touch is actually an understatement. These people are legit living on a different planet. We're not even real, flesh-and-blood human beings to them. We're just like passing faces in a crowd in their eyes—nothing but people-shaped cardboard cutouts.

I want to ask you about the media thing, because I think it's important for us to talk about that and document it here. In years to come, I wonder if we're even going to be able to remember what the situation was like for us during this year, how we got our news, how we communicated with each other, etc. I mean, if people weren't on social media before, the pandemic probably pushed them to get plugged in. For a lot of us that was the one way we could connect with one another or learn about what was going on in the world. And so, I wanted to ask what it was like for you and also your friends, boyfriend, coworkers, etc. when we went into lockdown and there was a lot of fear and uncertainty. How did y'all figure out what was happening elsewhere? Where did you turn to? What sources were you looking at to stay informed?

Ashley: I grew up when the internet came around, and I've watched the beautiful thing that the internet was turn into something totally different. The internet used to bring people together—you could see how people live and exist on other sides of the planet. You could learn about people like, "Oh, this person has a YouTube channel talking about what it's like to be trans. Oh, this person grew up as a hermaphrodite. What's that like? Oh, this person lives in a faraway country. How do they live?" You know what I mean? The internet has connected us in a lot of ways.

However, the past, I would say, seven year or so it's definitely pitted a lot of people against each other. Now it's all screaming into the void. You have no accountability because you're just yelling at a screen. This is why I'm actually not a huge social media user. My last boyfriend—he barely used social media, which is one of the things I found attractive about him. I saw how social media was ruining, like, the sacredness of my time. You don't ever get that time back. And I saw how it caused rifts among friends—that and fantasy football. Fantasy football has ruined friendships, too, I've noticed. But I will say that there was this blossoming, beautiful thing in the beginning of COVID that was bringing people together. The bartender community was doing something called "cocktail boomerangs" where you'd make five of a certain type of cocktail, then somebody would come pick them up and switch them all out with five new cocktails. People were giving each other shoutouts online, and some would post things explaining how they made these drinks . . . the tinctures, bitters, and everything else that went into it, etc. I didn't actually participate, but it was fun to follow that. It was nice to see people being like, "Even in these times of strife, you just gotta keep going, you gotta reinvent, and you make something new of it. This is not the time to just lie down and die."

Speaking of which, I was gonna mention this later, because it's really sad, but when we did reopen the first time—because that's the thing, there's actually been two lockdowns here so far—I would see my friends and their mental health was horrible. Horrible. Oh, and that reminds me of another point about social media. Like I said, I don't do a lot of social media. I would go on Instagram occasionally. And I have a Facebook, but I don't use it much. When I would go on Facebook, though, it was weird going through my feed and seeing both sides. Remember, I have lived in Portland and I've lived in Florida—these are two very, very different social settings [laughs]. It's funny to flick through your feed and you've got people like, "I'm out here with no mask! Take that, you stupid lib-tards!" Then you've got other people wearing masks and virtue signaling about it like, "Wear your masks! Stop being a conserva-twat!"

I will say, though, that social media was a really good avenue for some people to come together, especially single people or people living alone. I have a lot of single friends, and I'm currently single during this second lockdown. Think of how much worse a lockdown would be if social media didn't exist! You'd probably have way more suicides.

Max: It would be really, really tough. I really do think that people staying connected on social media played a big role in keeping society from totally crumbling. And I was just talking to a parent about this—I was asking her what it was like trying to raise kids during all this. Because I keep wondering . . . if something like COVID happened when we were growing up, before we had the internet or all these smartphones and tablets to connect us, what do you think we would have done? I don't even know.

Ashley: Yeah, me neither. I run the bar's social media, so I have to have it. Otherwise I'd probably delete my Facebook and my Instagram. I still like Reddit, though. During COVID, I would keep refreshing the Portland Reddit page and see what people were going through. That was a good avenue for me in the beginning of the shutdown. I could go on Reddit and be like, "Oh, this person's having a problem with unemployment. This is what they did. Oh, this place is still open. Hey, this store is out of this or that product." Reddit was very helpful as a community and a tool for knowing what the fuck was going on in a local sense. But there was also the thing where you'd see some people post on social media, then you'd see them in person, and those are two different things, you know? You'd see it, too—a lot of people wear their unhappiness on their outside. I watched so many people gain weight and lose weight. I almost felt bad because during the first lockdown, since I had a boyfriend, I had companionship. We would go backpacking all the time or go to the coast, I was trying out new recipes, etc. I was constantly busy during the first shutdown, trying to make the most of it. But when I would hang out with my friends I'd see how it was affecting people differently. A lot of my friends were very depressed. Very depressed.

Oh, that reminds me, I did want to say one more thing about the unemployment stuff. Never in my life have I gone on unemployment. If I've ever been let go or if I ever quit a job I just went and found a new job. I'm a very hardworking, capable person. But when this happened, immediately I was just like, "Oh, fuck. They're giving me *my* money that I've been paying into for forever. It's called *insurance*: unemployment insurance." I never thought I would feel that way. If it was a different time or place I feel like I would be embarrassed to be getting unemployment. I'd be telling myself to just pull myself up by my bootstraps, go get another job, etc. But, like, this is unprecedented, and I didn't feel ashamed at all. I was like, "No, give me my money back." That's kind of how I felt about it. And, like we were talking about, I was also shocked by how completely unprepared the government was to help all these people in need. I will say, though, that a lot of people who got unemployment were doing pretty okay with that extra $600. A friend of mine who is also a bartender and was also on unemployment brought this up the other day. Some people were getting their regular unemployment, which was like $200 to $500, plus $600 from the extended benefits for weeks. So, the government did help out in a certain way. I know people—and it was a very small percentage—who were making more money on unemployment for a while than from being employed. And good! Those people probably needed the money anyway. But yeah, there are so many other ways we got screwed over. Why couldn't we be like Canada and get even temporary Medicare for All? You can give us money and we'll all stay home! Give us the money to do that and we could contain this thing.

Max: Speaking of staying home, what has it been like since the second lockdown?

Ashley: Well, I'm single this lockdown. But, I mean, I got this cat. I got him while things were open for a while. He's a Sphynx. I've always wanted one of those. So I finally got my dream cat. But for the first two months, like a lot of people in my industry, I reverted back to my alcoholic ways. During the lockdowns I know a bunch of hospitality people were playing video games, jerking off, eating food, and getting drunk. I literally have seen some of my friends . . . like, that's what they do from the time they wake up to the time they go to bed: video games, jerk off, drink till you blackout, then do it again—and forget to shower. The first month that we were closed again I definitely went down a drinking hole. But . . . I don't know. One day I woke up and was just like, "Oh, I'm a fucking loser right now. I don't want to be a loser anymore." So I decided to make a change. I've always been interested in building websites and stuff, and I've dabbled with coding on and off for years, but I was just like, "Man, I've always talked about doing a coding bootcamp. I know that a four-year degree is not for me. I know that if I learn some skills I can get a job in tech. I've been talking about it for years, so I'm just gonna do that." And so, I quit drinking a while ago, I make sure I work out every day, and I'm enrolled in a program that starts on February 1.

I think there does have to be some accountability for people and their own well-being. And I'm not . . . I don't know . . . I guess my point is: Your government's not there for you, so we have to take care of ourselves. Also, you can't get a therapist anywhere right now. I've tried. I'm sure I should try harder, but every place I've called has said the same thing: "We're not accepting new patients," "We're not accepting new patients," "We're not accepting new patients." Like pretty much the rest of America I have anxiety and depression and, honestly, I had always been against prescriptions for mental illness, but I think if I hadn't got onto Wellbutrin two years ago I might be in a really different place right now. Wellbutrin changed things for me drastically.

Max: Man, I've talked to so many people who have had the same difficulty trying to find a therapist this past year, right when they needed it most. And it really makes me think . . . How can we even try to calculate the sheer mental weight of all of this? It's impossible. I honestly don't know what we're all going to be like coming out of it—how the things we've experienced and the memories we'll carry with us will continue to shape us. That's why I don't think that we're ever going to be able to just go "back to normal" when we're vaccinated. Not to mention the fact that wealthy countries like the U.S. have hoarded vaccines and fucked over billions of people around the world, which means that countless more people dying while we get vaccinated every year for new COVID strains *is* the new normal. We may try to make society feel as normal as possible after this, but we won't be the same people, and I wonder how that's gonna manifest in how we live and think. Because we can't unsee what we've seen. We can't unlearn what this pandemic taught us about ourselves and our society. From the painful isolation and lack of social connection to the many ways our government and the market just abandoned us, to the shitty ways our bosses and customers treated us . . . all those experiences are gonna leave an imprint. So many folks I've talked to over the past year have said some version of the same thing: "The pandemic showed working people how little our lives are actually worth to this system." Millionaire politicians refusing to give people the aid we needed, business owners telling us on TV to go work and die "for the economy," even our neighbors and customers treating us like disposable human beings—refusing to follow safety protocols where people work, assaulting flight attendants for enforcing mask wearing, etc.—we saw how vicious and unjust our society can become when the chips are down. Doesn't inspire much hope for how we'll deal with climate catastrophe, to be honest. So, how do you move on from that? How do you "go back to normal" and carry on participating in a society you've lost so much faith in?

But this is also why it's so important to highlight the good that we saw in each other this past year, because that's what got us through. There've been really incredible stories of people banding together, people supporting one another, taking care of each other, and people finding creative ways to be together. And there have also been great stories of jobs *not* abandoning their workers. Like you said, you're fortunate enough to work at a place that you ike with a boss you like, and there were other businesses that prioritized workers' safety, etc. So hopefully we can take some valuable lessons away from that. I don't know . . . I guess it depends on what day of the week you ask me. I tend to seesaw between hope and despair. But I do think that the emotional strain and the psychological strain that this has put on so many of us—that's gonna linger for a long time.

Ashley: Yeah. We opened for a brief time during the summer and it was really nice to see all the regulars, and they were so happy to see me, and you got all those pity tips for being unemployed for so long. But there's also that weird look they give you like, "Are you okay?" And I'm like, "Are *you* okay?"

I know a lady who's a nurse and she has two little four-year-old girls—they're twins—and she stopped by during that brief time between lockdowns. She was going off about how kids are gonna be so fucked up because they're in these important developmental years when they're supposed to be learning to read facial expressions, but because of the lockdown they're not gonna learn to read facial expressions as easily as a child that grew up in a different period. My other friend has a two-year-old and, you know, other parents don't want them to play together unless they're in some kind of learning pod. So, yeah, kids are gonna be real weird for a couple years.

This is why I really don't like the phrase "return to normal." Everyone says, "Oh, I just want to go back to normal!" Yeah, well, that's not a thing. That's not happening. I don't feel like there's any "going back" to "normal." There might be a return to normal in the sense that the economy will be really booming by the end of this year, I think—maybe next spring. But I think there's also going to be more governmental control in your life, your taxes are probably going to be higher, health care is still going to suck, etc.

Max: I could talk to you about this for days, but I don't want to keep you too long. By way of rounding us out, let's fill out the rest of the timeline here. You were saying that you guys went into lockdown back in March, then the governor kind of flip-flopped, reopened things, then there was another shutdown in the summer . . .

Ashley: So, we had that first lockdown and it was hard for a lot of people, but it was also in the summer so a lot of people were still hanging out at parks. I was kind of enjoying the three-month break. But my boss also tried to do takeout and cheapened his menu. He was like, "Well, we're a neighborhood bar. I want to make things affordable and keep people employed." He tried to do that, but we were just in a weird spot—we're not really known for our food. So that didn't work, unfortunately. Then he got the PPP loan, so we opened back up, everybody came back. He spent so much money trying to get ready for the winter, like building a patio area, getting tents, buying heaters. Also, our menu used to be all over the place—it was more like American bar food, I guess. But my boss went to his Korean roots and made a whole new menu based on his family's recipes. That was a cool change, but that also took a lot of money, you know? New menus, new product, training all of our employees again, etc. You saw so many businesses like ours trying to do so much, then we all just got locked down again. We were open for about three months before the second lockdown started in November . . . it came on November 18, which is my birthday, so it's easy for me to remember. And before the second lockdown all these businesses, including ours, were trying everything they could. It was like, "Yes, we're making everyone wear masks. Yes, we're sanitizing behind and between each thing every chance we get."

So, in all honesty, when this lockdown happened I was glad for it. I wasn't like, "Oh, I'm happy to just sit at home and collect a government check" like you hear these stupid Republicans talking about. It's more because working at that point was terrible. It was the worst time I've ever spent bartending. I'm currently the only front-of-house employee who's coming back to the bar whenever we reopen, because my coworkers couldn't do it anymore. They were just like, "Nah, we're gonna go find new shit to do. We can't do this." They said bartending wasn't fun anymore. For example, there's a nice restaurant up the road where your bill for a meal is gonna be, like, a couple hundred bucks. Their servers and bartenders would come down to our bar after they got off the clock and they would try to come in without masks. And I'm like, "Dude, you just got off work where you and your customers were wearing masks—why are you disrespecting me and coming in here right now not wearing a mask?" And the regulars would have too many drinks then try to walk around without a mask. And when I'd be like, "Sir, pull up your mask," I'd get people saying, "Well, don't you think that violates my civil liberties?" "No, sir. I don't. And there are people waiting behind you." Everyone wanted to argue constantly and not wear a mask. It just got so frustrating and it would wear on you—you would go into work in a good mood, but by five o'clock your stress level was so high. It's just . . . I was happy for the bar to close. And I never thought I would say something like that. Now that I've had two months off I'm like, "I gotta go back to work." But working during COVID was just so insanely stressful that it was actually a relief when that second lockdown happened.

Max: It's especially sad, too, because you were saying earlier that one of your favorite parts about working at this bar before the pandemic—and the very reason so many of the regulars were always coming back—was that social aspect, right? Not to sound too hokey about it, but from what you described it sounded like a place where people felt more at home, where people knew each other, where you could get into conversations with Ashley, your friendly neighborhood bartender. Then to see the COVID version of that where everyone is stressed, where people are being dicks and trying to make some dumb fucking point about not wearing a mask, where people are saying really vicious things to each other—it's just really sad. It seems like what happened at your bar was emblematic of this larger disintegration of the social fabric that I think we've all seen and experienced across the country.

Ashley: Yeah. And physically, I mean, my hands were *wrecked*. I was constantly touching money and washing my hands after. Because we have those lotto machines and we're a neighborhood bar where people like to pay with cash, so we can't just go cashless. And then, like I said, just dealing with people was very exhausting. Luckily, a lot of people did sit outside, which was a blessing and a curse, because on one hand I didn't have to deal with some of the more annoying customers, but on the other hand it kind of sucked because people couldn't just sit at the bar and bullshit with me while I do my thing. That was kind of a bummer. And even with the customers who were really frustrating, it's just . . . people are people, and these aren't bad people. They're just not as aware as they should be, especially when they've had a few drinks, and I get it. But it's disheartening, and it was just so frustrating. I'm hoping that, once we're out of this lockdown, people will maybe have their shit together.

10. Mx. Pucks A'Plenty

I am Mx. Pucks A'Plenty. I am a burlesque performer, producer, sex worker, and sex educator based out of Seattle, Washington.

Max: Well, Mx. Pucks, it is wonderful to talk to you, thank you so much for making time to do this. I'm really excited to get to know more about you, your life, your work, and how you have been navigating this very wild year that we've all been through. Before we get to all that, though, let's start small: Are you originally from Seattle?

Mx. Pucks: Yup, born and raised, which is actually kind of rare these days. Seattle is definitely more of a transient sort of place now with the Amazons and the Googles. There are a lot of Amazon bros out here . . . There are a lot of transplants in Seattle. In my social circle I think I'm probably one of three folks who are actually born-and-raised Washingtonians.

Max: Wow. What was it like seeing that change happen? Not to put you on the spot or anything, I'm just really curious because this is something I think about a lot. I grew up in Southern California, and in a weird way we have a similar problem. Like Florida, Southern California is where everyone goes when they finally get fed up with winters in the Midwest and stuff, right? So you have all these transplants who end up becoming like SoCal natives by proxy. That's always been a regular part of the landscape back home. But I guess that's why it feels a little different when you compare it to places like Seattle, because it was a pretty common, pretty constant feature of living there, even for people who were born and raised there like me. Plenty of "native" Southern Californians aren't originally from there [laughs]. What did Seattle look like when you were growing up? When did you notice that Seattle itself started changing into what it is now?

Mx. Pucks: Seattle has always been this kind of odd liberal beacon. We have this "Anything goes in Seattle" reputation, which I think partly came from early '90s with grunge music. So people associate living out here with this alternative lifestyle. It's assumed that folks are just a little different here. And there are a lot of great things about Seattle, to be fair. There's so many bars and so many music venues, and it's such an artistic place— there's theaters everywhere, performance art everywhere. I would say that it was probably around the early 2000s when things started to look a little different. Honestly, it's really been in the past, like, eight to ten years that it's changed a lot—like night and day. We were losing venues . . . music venues, art venues . . . *before* COVID hit. COVID really just knocked some of the other ones off that had been holding on by the skin of their teeth.

There's a specific neighborhood, the Capitol Hill neighborhood of Seattle, that became very popular this past summer because of the CHOP [Capitol Hill Organized Protest][8] and all that. That neighborhood—that was the gay neighborhood. That was where all the art was happening, that was where you went to get the coolest clothes, that was where you went out on Friday and Saturday night. That was the place to be. But it has slowly become gentrified and it's pretty alarming. And the neighborhood that kind of sits on top of that is called the Central District of Seattle. The Central District was a historically Black neighborhood. In the past decade, though, most of the Black and Brown folks who lived there have all been shoved out. And they really love those ugly, boxy townhouses over there too. They're so ugly and they look exactly the same. It's like a townhouse setup with three floors and there's a bedroom on each floor, you know? So those are sprouting up everywhere in the Central District. And it's really interesting to watch some of the White folks who have moved into this historically Black neighborhood, because they look at the people of color there as if *they're* misplaced, like *they* shouldn't be there. It's really sad.

---

8 The Capitol Hill Organized Protests (CHOP) began on June 8, 2020, as part of the mass protests that spread throughout the U.S.—and beyond—in the wake of Minneapolis police officer Derek Chauvin murdering George Floyd on May 26. After Seattle Police Department staff evacuated the East Precinct building in Capitol Hill in response to the demonstrations, protestors established the surrounding area, spanning six blocks and Cal Anderson Park, as the Capitol Hill Autonomous Zone (CHAZ), which they successfully occupied and operated communally until police eventually cleared the area on July 1.

My great-grandmother had a house in the Central District when I was a kid, and that house was actually on sale recently, about five months ago. I went to look at it just out of curiosity, but also because I was thinking, "Maybe, if I can pull my crap together, I could get my great-grandma's house back." They wanted like $700,000 for that house! And the house was on the market for less than a week. Now someone's gonna tear that house down and put something else up, because that's what they're doing everywhere. And it's just . . . it's depressing. As it is, Seattle *before* COVID was already getting to be pretty depressing. We have homeless folks everywhere and all people want to do is throw them in jail, force them to get clean, force them to do whatever, and it's just awful. That's not how it should be. And, again, folks always hold Seattle up as this intensely liberal beacon, even though it has done the most harm to its most marginalized people . . . It's pretty frustrating.

Max: It is incredibly frustrating, even just on the surface of it. But then if you add that personal attachment, especially for someone like you, having grown up there, having family roots there, having seen the city change, and having felt—I have to imagine—so powerless against the onslaught of that change . . . I can only imagine how frustrating it is. It's like trying to hold water in your hands.

Mx. Pucks: Mmhmm.

Max: I mean, that story about your great-grandma's house just breaks my heart. What can you do when the property value is so ridiculously high? Anyone who isn't a wealthy investor looking to build some new fucking condos is just going to be priced out completely.

I wanted to ask a little more about the way things used to be, because I'm really curious to know how you fit into all of this. You talked about grunge and the art scene. So, like, were you a "scene" kid? Were you going to these artsy dive places, going to gigs, and all that? And speaking of scenes . . . is there a big burlesque tradition in Seattle?

Mx. Pucks: Um, I was a pretty straightlaced kid. Even into my early twenties I was pretty straightlaced. Going out clubbing wasn't really my scene.

But I do love dancing, so every once in a while someone could convince me to go out dancing. But I'm kind of an old lady at heart [laughs]. I'm the designated driver. Whenever we're out somewhere, I'm always the one person who doesn't want to go to the second location. Someone will be like, "Oh, let's go to this other bar!" And I'm like, "Nah."

Max: [Laughs.] Hey, man, every crew needs one . . .

Mx. Pucks: [Laughs.] Exactly. It's like, "Nope! We're not going, sorry." But, yeah, when it comes to the burlesque scene, burlesque here in Seattle is pretty fantastic. Neo-burlesque is basically what everyone's doing right now. And Seattle and New York are considered, like, the figureheads of the neo-burlesque resurgence back in the late '90s. Seattle is home to two previous Miss Exotic World titleholders, which is the biggest honor you can get in burlesque. There's also a restaurant-bar here called The Pink Door, and when you go down to The Pink Door you'll see painted across the building this giant mural of a burlesque performer named Waxie Moon. Seattle loves its burlesque—loves it, loves it, loves it. And the roots of burlesque here are amazing too. We have an area in Seattle called Pioneer Square, for example, and that was basically like our Skid Row, but it's where all the burlesque was happening. That's where all the gay clubs were, that was where you went to have a little more spicy of a late-night experience back in, like, the late 1800s, early 1900s, down there in Pioneer Square.

Burlesque is kind of folded into the fabric of Seattle, even though it doesn't get as much respect as an art form as I think it should. And the cool thing about burlesque . . . well, it's cool to me, at least . . . is that burlesque has its origins in being a political art form. Burlesque was used to kind of poke fun at the aristocrats, the rich folks, and all of that. They used it to make fun of all the morals of the day. And it was just wonderfully ribald— there was stripping, there was comedy, and sideshow. It was kind of this thing that you did so you could see the world in a different way, something that made it a little bit easier to digest the ridiculous nature of the politics of the time. Also, like, whatever time period you're in, when you have women or female-identified folks on stage taking off their clothes it becomes political, because folks think that they have control over femme bodies. Femme bodies are typically seen as some man's possession or some product for sale. It's like we don't really have ownership over our own bodies. So it's a very intense political statement when a femme-presenting person gets on stage and takes off their clothes to some music and they're covered in glitter—it's a statement. Even if they're in an overly ornate costume and it's gorgeous, and there's an orchestra in the background and all of that, it's still a political statement. I think that's what drew me, personally, to burlesque.

Max: Damn. That's *such* an interesting history—and, I'll admit, it's one that I'm very fascinated by but know very little about. I wanted to ask a little more about this, if that's okay, because when you said that burlesque has its origins as a political art form that really struck me. I thought that was a really compelling way to put it, and now I'm over here thinking about all the different ways that burlesque, like you said, has this rich history of being a space, being an art form, that kind of flips the norms and power arrangements of society on their head. And there are a lot of layers to that too, right? A few years back, I remember reading somewhere that night clubs and burlesque scenes in places like New York and Chicago were not only places where folks would sort of flip the script on gender power dynamics, but they were also places where different races would congregate and flout racial hierarchies and all that stuff. It's clear you know a lot about this history and you have a deep passion for it, so could you talk a little more about that history and that political tradition of burlesque? Also, I'm really curious to know what it was like for you, personally, to get drawn into burlesque, to get so invested in that history, and to become part of that tradition . . .

Mx. Pucks: My journey to getting involved in burlesque was a long one. I have a kiddo . . . my kiddo is eleven . . . and right after I had my child I was going through postpartum depression. It was just a really stressful time. And I remember one day I was nursing my kid and surfing Netflix, trying to find something to watch, and I found this documentary called *A Wink and a Smile*, which has a little bit on burlesque history, but it also talks about a modern-day Academy of Burlesque. I was like, "Oh, so there's actually an Academy of Burlesque that exists out in the world where people can go and take these classes." It turns out that particular academy from the documentary happens to be in Seattle . . . So, I was watching this documentary and I was just enthralled. Like I said, it gives you a little history of burlesque, but it also transports you into this thing called "Burlesque 101" here in Seattle. It's like a six-week intensive burlesque course where they help you create an act, then you perform the act at a recital for your family and friends. And in the documentary you get to see the journey of these students in this class, and you get to see how burlesque kind of transforms them. Like, it made folks more confident, it made folks accept their bodies, it made them feel powerful and accomplished. It's beautiful. And, again, as someone who just had a baby and was going through postpartum depression, that kind of empowerment was very intriguing to me.

After that I started going to one burlesque show a year in Seattle. It was like a once-a-year treat to myself. And that particular burlesque show, the one I would watch once a year, is kind of like the top-tier of what you can see out there. So I'm watching it like, "Oh, I don't know how to do ballet, I don't know what's going on here. I can't do this." But I loved watching it. And so I decided to look and see how much it would cost to go to this Academy of Burlesque, but every time I did I'd come up with some excuse for why I couldn't go, why we couldn't spend the money. About three and a half years ago, though, I was tasked with creating a fundraiser for an organization in Seattle called the Center for Sex Positive Culture, and they wanted to do a cabaret fundraising show. We planned it out, and a good friend of mine was like, "I know burlesque dancers," and I'm like, "Cool, let's bring some in." And I just remember this group of folks they brought in—they were so fun, hilarious, and super sexy, and they had their own shared lingo. And to me it just seemed like this is a really fun world to be in. We ended up doing a second show and I remember afterward the burlesquers in that show were just like, "You really should do burlesque. You should take a class. You should do it." So I finally got up the courage, did a drop-in class, and really loved it. After that I found the money to take the "Burlesque 101" class, and at the time I thought, "Okay, I'll take the class, I'll get it out of my system, then I'll be done." Three and a half years later, I have performed in over six burlesque festivals, including one international festival. I've produced two burlesque festivals myself. I run an arts organization called Puckduction and we produce at least six or seven burlesque shows a year, and I've gotten to teach as well. It's really opened up a whole lot of doors.

When we talk about burlesque being political . . . that's really what drove me to it in the first place. My very first burlesque act was to En Vogue's "Free Your Mind," which is about racial discrimination—it ends with me wearing a hoodie that says "Black Lives Matter" on the back and I've got my hands up in the air. Every time we do this act I always tell every lighting person and tech person I work with, "It's very important to me that, when you see that happen, you change the lights to blue and red, because I want it to look like the cops have shown up." So, my very first act was this political statement about my Blackness. And I think that is where I find my home in burlesque. Black femmes are told that we can't really be much of anything. My friend says that Black femmes are not meant to be the protagonists of their own stories. I firmly believe that we live in a society where Black femmes are supposed to help everyone else achieve what they need to achieve, and then we're supposed to just go away. Doing burlesque allows me to be the hero of my own stories, of my own art.

There's all kinds of fun stuff that happens in burlesque too! Burlesque, especially modern burlesque, takes a lot of its love and a lot of its artistry from drag—and drag is *extremely* political, right? You have a lot of gender-bending happening in burlesque, and there's *a lot* of queer folks. I would say that if you go to a burlesque show and there are ten femme burlesque performers, 80 percent of those ladies are not interested in any penis-having individual in the room, because they are either lesbians or bisexuals who only put up with dudes when they have to [laughs]. And there's a pretty fascinating history behind that too, which has its roots in, like, burlesque back in the '30s and '40s. A lot of those women who were doing burlesque back then, I mean, think about it . . . back then, to be a stripper, to decide that's what you're going to do, immediately puts you on the fringes of society. You're saying that you're not going to have a husband, because you're traveling across the country. A lot of those women—their families had abandoned them, or they left home from abusive families, or they left home because this is what they wanted to do. And a lot of them were lesbians—that was a safe (or *safer*) place for them to be. The women who held the suitcases for these glamorous burlesque ladies—they used to call them "suitcase butches." They could have their own money and have control over their own lives. To be a burlesque performer was to basically be on this path of financial security for yourself and financial control for yourself. And, especially when we get into the '50s and '60s, that was just unheard of. People would just look at you like, "What are you doing? You should have a husband, you should be at home."

This also becomes a very fascinating story for performers of color too. Some of the shows back then were heavily segregated of course. But there were also a lot of things that old-school burlesques used to do that would have us all clutching our pearls now. There were a lot of White women who basically did black-, brown-, and yellow-face to be more exotic. There was a lot of cultural appropriation with, like, belly dancing and dressing up like geishas, and there were *a lot* of indigenous headdresses, especially in the '60s and stuff—it was really intense. That was their artistic expression. What's really fascinating, though, is that now, in the burlesque community, we really honor those legends. We have folks who were out here doing it for a really long time, folks who are in their eighties now, and they're honored every year. The Burlesque Hall of Fame in Las Vegas does a "Legends Night," so these women will come out—and they're in their seventies and eighties—and do burlesque, and it's beautiful. It's also kind of haunting in a way. Because you realize, like . . . it never leaves you. Once a performer, always a performer. And I just, I don't know . . . I want to be seventy-five humping a curtain on stage, and my son will be in the audience like, "That's my mon! That's what they're doing today" [Laughs.] Something about that is really wonderful and really interesting. And burlesque is a very feminist art form, especially now, which, again, makes it very political. I would say that more than half of the productions that are happening out here in burlesque are femme-run—it's probably closer to three-fourths. Men who are involved in burlesque are a guest in someone's house, you know? So, from the beginnings all the way to now, it's very political.

Max: That's really incredible. And like you said, just having that sense of tradition . . . it's such a powerful thing. Once you feel it, you never forget it. Once you feel it, you realize how much of you was missing before when you didn't know about it. I guess, going back to the discussion we were having at the beginning about the places we grow up in and how they're hollowed out by gentrification, it's like there are so many histories and traditions we're not really allowed to become attached to in this country because "progress" erases them and paves them over with concrete. In so many big and little ways, we're denied that kind of connection to tradition. But when you find it in places like these, when you celebrate it, when you feel part of it, it's indescribable. And you realize just how much you need it, how much you miss it, and how cruel it is that we're denied it with such frequency.

Mx. Pucks: There's gotta be a way to be able to hold space for our history, while understanding that things change. I'm very into, like, woo-woo, connecting with your ancestors, and all of that. Because these stories—they have to live on somewhere. We've gotta keep telling the stories. And a lot of our history, especially for people of color, was oral, right? A lot of our history lives in oral traditions and dance and music. That's the beauty of it. Our history is . . . it's *there*, and it's never going to go away. It lives on through us, through our music, our movements, through dancing, the stories we tell. Being able to honor those traditions is really important. And sure, progress happens, things are gonna change, but I think it's important to never forget where you come from.

Max: Mmhmm. Man, that's really beautifully put. And this makes me think about that first act that you did in burlesque, which, like you said, was a very political performance. I wanted to ask about that, and about what burlesque has meant for how you connect to those larger traditions of race, ethnicity, and identity. Because every person of color has their own story about this, right? And you're clearly telling a story with that performance. What role has burlesque played for you when it comes to navigating your own racial identity? Did burlesque provide an outlet for you to express thoughts, feelings, and critiques about race that had been simmering somewhere inside you? Or was it more of a situation where getting into burlesque kind of unlocked a lot of thoughts and feelings and reflections on race in society you didn't know you had? Does that question make sense?

Mx. Pucks: It does, yeah. I think it was more that I felt like, "I need to tell these stories. These stories need to be told." And what a disarming way to tell the story, right? You're thinking, "I'm going to a titty show." Then it's a Black Lives Matter burlesque act and you're like, "Well, fuck . . . cool . . . [laughs] now I have that to think about." And so, for me it was all about, "*How* do I tell these stories? These are stories that need to be told, but how do I tell them in a way that feels authentic—and authentic *to me*?" Because I have ideas all the time, but sometimes I'll think, "That's not my lived experience, so I don't really need to tell that story."

Another burlesque act that I have is called "Colorism in A-Minor," and it's done to a Postmodern Jukebox version of the song "Creep" by Radiohead. It's a really gorgeous version of the song. The whole act is about skin bleaching. So, under my wig we created these fake skin-bleaching spots, and they're on my arms too, which are covered with gloves. When I do the glove peel you see the uneven skin bleaching that is happening. It's a really powerful piece, because it's a classic burlesque piece, but it's horrifying. The whole time you're seeing my reaction to not having the bleach cover my whole skin and you're seeing the depression of it. And there's always White people in the audience, right? So what typically happens in this act is I'm looking at my skin, and I'm looking back at them. I point to their skin, or I reach out to them, and it becomes really uncomfortable and oddly personal, and it makes people stop and think. It's a mindfuck. I am a kinkster first and foremost—BDSM is my jam. One of my favorite things about BDSM is power exchange—I love mindfucking people. And that's part of the magic, especially with this act—making White people feel really uncomfortable about this thing that is very common in Africa and also places like Korea. They sell a lot of skin-bleaching stuff in Korea. And they should be uncomfortable, because colorism is so damaging. This act is one of my favorite acts. And, like I said, it's a very classic act—it could fit into any really beautiful burlesque show, except that it has this extremely horrifying element to it. And that element is something that really affects people of color—this idea of Whiteness being rightness.

Max: Damn, that's incredibly powerful—wish I could see that live. And it makes me wonder about folks who are reading this, folks who maybe have never been to a burlesque before, or who have only thought about burlesque, perhaps, as it's portrayed in pop culture. This will all probably sound a little shocking to them, right? Maybe they're expecting burlesque to be like strip clubs in a theater setting—or something like that. I dunno. And I love how you're playing with those misguided expectations in your act. You're turning them into something you can use in the act itself. For instance, you said something that really caught my ear when you were talking about how straight, cisgender men are guests in this space. But so much of what we expect burlesques to be is still filtered through that cis, straight male gaze, you know? I have to imagine that for a lot of readers, they're probably assuming that you go to a burlesque for a very specific reason. As an audience member, you're maybe expecting, I dunno, a sexy show with half-naked women that is meant to provide you with some sort of gratification. What you're describing is very different. There probably isn't one definitive answer to this, but for readers who are unfamiliar with this world I wanted to ask: What is the space of burlesque for? And *who* is it for?

Mx. Pucks: Okay, so this is really interesting. Because, yes, what you see in pop culture and in the media is very much filtered through that male gaze. Most folks who've never even been to a burlesque show before can probably name only one burlesque performer, because she's got a really good marketing machine, and that's Dita Von Teese. Everyone knows that Dita Von Teese is a burlesque performer, even if you don't really know what burlesque is. And Dita Von Teese has a very specific type of look, but burlesque across the country doesn't necessarily have that particular look.

First of all, burlesque is really queer—it's very, very queer. But also, burlesque is big money when it's really in that classic style—big, big money. A lot of burlesque performers are on what we call the "corporate gigs." When someone wants to throw a splashy party at a hotel they bring in three or four burlesque performers, and they come with their giant feather fans and their beautiful boas, and it's all very sexy and very classic. Then you go to burlesques in other parts of the country and it's very different. Here in Seattle, for instance, we have a really beautiful venue called The Rendezvous. It's a really cute, small venue, and you'll see classic burlesque there, but you'll also see what they call "nerdlesque." Nerdlesque is like the intersection of burlesque and cosplay, and it's *amazing*. I was part of a show once that was all Marvel stuff, so I have a "Women of Wakanda" act.

Max: Nice!

Mx. Pucks: There's been *tons* of Harry Potter burlesque shows too. There's a *Jurassic Park* burlesque show that's happening soon. It's wild. Nerdlesque is so, so fun. Here in Seattle, someone recently did a *Muppet Show* burlesque show . . .

Max: [Laughs.] That's awesome.

Mx. Pucks: Right? So, it's stuff like that—really heavily themed, really fun. I did a burlesque show that was all John Hughes movies—*everything* had to be related to a John Hughes movie—and that was called "The Burly Pack." We had a *Pretty in Pink* act, *The Breakfast Club*, someone did an act from the first *Family Vacation* movie, which I totally forgot was a John Hughes movie [laughs]. It was pretty great. There's this really nerdy, fun element that happens with some of these themed shows.

So burlesque is everything that you think it is and absolutely not at all what you think it is all in the same breath. I ran a show for a venue in Seattle for over a year, and we'd bring in three burlesque performers who would do two acts each. Sometimes the stuff was so ridiculous and silly and avant-garde, but other times it was, like, super-duper classic. We tried to really mix it up and give folks an idea of what they could see at other burlesque shows. I like to tell folks that there is a burlesque show out there for everyone—there really is. Maybe you're thinking, "Well, I'm a mathematician. There's absolutely nothing out there for me." Well, a really good friend of mine produced a show called "SCIENCE." Every single burlesque performer in that show was working in a STEM field, and everything was very science-based—hilarious and sexy and fun, but still rooted in science. And that show was standing room only! There's literally something for everyone.

When it comes to audience expectations, I mean, if you are a person who can't keep your hands to yourself burlesque is probably not a place you should be going to. To be honest, you probably shouldn't be going anywhere if you're not able to keep your hands to yourself—you should probably just stay home and work on that. That's one of the things I really like about burlesque. Pretty much every burlesque show that I've been a part of . . . especially live burlesque shows . . . the hosts always have a mini conversation about consent with the audience, and it's great. Stuff like, "Don't touch the performers. If the performer is interested in touching you they will give you a clear indication that that's what's going to happen." And if you're not interested in participating, usually we will give the audience a signal that they can use to let the performers know they're not interested in being part of the act. So the audience gets that crash course in consent right at the beginning of the show and it really kind of sets the mood. I feel like I have heard more conversations about consent in burlesque than in most other spaces that I'm a part of. And I'm heavily involved in the kink scene—we talk about consent all the time. But burlesque performers talk about it *a lot*. It's pretty great.

Max: So, as you know, a big chunk of the conversations we're having for this book focuses on work and our working lives. From watching that documentary on Netflix about the Academy of Burlesque all the way to now, was there a particular moment for you when you decided to kind of thrust yourself into burlesque as a career? And could we talk about the work aspect of burlesque? What is it like to be a worker in burlesque? Like, what goes into a "typical week" for you? Before the pandemic, that is . . . I guess there's nothing "typical" about how we've been living and working the past year. And, again, just to make sure that readers are up to speed, how is burlesque connected to the sex industry . . . are they connected?

Mx. Pucks: They are. And I think it's disingenuous when I hear burlesque performers say things like, "We're not strippers." I laugh at that—I laugh really hard. Also, what's wrong with being a stripper? "But what *we* do is called striptease." No, you're fooling yourselves. I would say that strippers working in a club work a lot harder than I do. Strippers have to be good at customer service. With all the face-to-face interactions, like, that's customer service and sales, and that's hard. I have a sales background—I don't even know how they do it. And they've got to dance on top of that, and they've got to constantly keep their body ready for that, right? Doing pole . . . you gotta be *strong*.

Max: Yeah!

Mx. Pucks: Someone accused me of being a pole dancer once. And I was just like, "Bless you. Bless you, sweet thing." [Laughs.] No way. I have terrible upper body strength—can't do it.

Max: Yeah, I can do approximately *two* pull-ups [laughs].

Mx. Pucks: [Laughs.] The funny thing is she meant it as this complete dis, but I was just like, "Bless you, child." Burlesque and traditional club stripping—they share a lot of roots. A lot of the neo-burlesque stars from the late '90s and early 2000s got their starts in strip clubs and peep shows, and they'll be the first to tell you. And a lot of them got into burlesque because they wanted to do these acts that were funny and silly and weird—acts that would not play in a strip club [laughs]. They'd be like, "Nope, we're not gonna let you just sit on a bunch of cakes at the strip club. Sorry, that's not happening."

Max: [Laughs.] You telling me they don't do Howard Hughes routines in the strip club?

Mx. Pucks: [Laughs.] Right? It's hilarious. Like I said, when neo-burlesque was really starting to kick off a lot of these burlesque folks were working in the club, and a lot of them were sex workers. Burlesque was more of a hobby for them, an outlet to do something a little bit different from what they would be able to do in a traditional strip club. So yeah, I would say that there is a lot of crossover between strippers and burlesque, and then there is some crossover into sex work too. Honestly, if nothing else taught us that, the passing of FOSTA-SESTA[9] sure did. In the eyes of this law bur-

---

9   The Stop Enabling Sex Traffickers Act (SESTA) and the Allow States and Victims to Fight Online Sex Trafficking Act (FOSTA), commonly referred to together as FOSTA-SESTA, are the U.S. House and Senate bills that were passed with overwhelming bipartisan support and signed into law by president Donald Trump on April 11, 2018. The bills were hailed by advocacy groups and politicians on both sides of the aisle as a victory for victims of sex trafficking and a major advance in the fight to curb illegal sex trafficking. However, free speech advocates and sex workers alike have decried the chilling and even draconian effects of the passage of FOSTA-SESTA. As Aja Roman, writing for *Vox*, sums it up, "the bills also poke a huge hole in a famous and longstanding 'safe harbor' rule of the internet: Section 230 of

lesque is considered adult entertainment. And it was frustrating to watch burlesque babes just kind of lose their shit and cry when it was passed, saying things like, "But we're not sex workers! We're not like them." That's the wrong response. We should be protecting our sisters in arms. If they go after them, they're gonna come after us when they're done with them. Trying to create that solidarity between the sex-positive art forms and sex-positive industries is kind of what I've fallen into doing.

When I first got into burlesque the idea really was that I needed something—I needed a hobby. I needed an outlet that wasn't being some person's mother, that wasn't just being someone's wife. I needed something that was for me. And so, what started off as a hobby became, "Well, I'm performing a couple nights a week now. Okay." And at the time I'm looking around, seeing different shows, and realizing that the shows aren't very diverse. I was like, "Oh, I could produce a show and cast predominantly people of color. I guess I'll do that." Before I knew it, it became a job—I was constantly doing burlesque stuff. On a typical day for me I wake up between 7:30 and 8 a.m., and the first thing I do is check my email and check Facebook, because we do a good chunk of our promotion through Facebook and Instagram. I'm my own admin most of the time—I handle all

the 1996 Communications Decency Act. Usually shorthanded as 'Section 230' and generally seen as one of the most important pieces of internet legislation ever created, it holds that 'No provider or user of an interactive computer service shall be treated as the publisher or speaker of any information provided by another information content provider.' In other words, Section 230 has allowed the internet to thrive on user-generated content without holding platforms and ISPs responsible for whatever those users might create. But FOSTA-SESTA creates an exception to Section 230 that means website publishers would be responsible if third parties are found to be posting ads for prostitution—including consensual sex work—on their platforms. The goal of this is supposed to be that policing online prostitution rings gets easier. What FOSTA-SESTA has actually done, however, is create confusion and immediate repercussions among a range of internet sites as they grapple with the ruling's sweeping language." Those immediate repercussions involved the loss of websites like Backpage, which sex workers had previously been able to use to advertise and engage in consensual sex work, while also being able to vet customers and protect their identities in the process. As numerous sex workers and allies argued before and after the passing of FOSTA-SESTA, eliminating these platforms that sex workers use to conduct their work as safely as they can won't eliminate sex work as such; it just forces sex workers to work under more dangerous conditions. "I would say that the passage of FOSTA-SESTA turned my world upside down," renowned author, educator, and phone-sex operator Jessie Sage told *City Paper* in Pittsburgh. "It made sex work less safe, especially for the most marginalized sex workers, and deplatformed all of us." Moreover, with websites scrambling to protect themselves from the sweeping language in FOSTA-SESTA by shutting down such pages and platforms, recent studies suggest the bills have actually made it *harder* to locate trafficking victims and identify trafficking transactions.

the social media. So, you're doing a lot with social media, a lot of promotion, then you have these contracts with different producers that specify what they want from you when you promote their show, so you have to make sure you go over those. And then, because I produce burlesques, a lot of that production work involves checking in and making sure I got all the contracts from performers for my show. If I've paid for ad space I've got to make sure that it's cleared, that I got the invoice, that the invoice gets put where it needs to go, etc. Also, my production company is fiscally sponsored, so it's like, "Okay, we got donations. I need to make sure the thank-you letters go out. Now I need to check ticket sales and make sure that's all good." And then there's costuming. I don't do a lot of it on my own—I'm not good at it. I mean, I can put rhinestones on things [laughs], but that's about it. So I've got to check in and make sure that what I've ordered is on its way. I've got to send in measurements and make sure that things are lining up where they need to line up. The work is constant: I can go into my home office at 9 a.m. and not come out until six. It's a full day of doing stuff and it's exhausting, but I like it. On top of that, I don't really have a day off—it's all day, every day. I'm probably talking about burlesque during all waking hours. The word "burlesque" probably leaves my mouth once every forty-five minutes at least, because it's just shaped my life so much. The majority of my really good friends that I've made in burlesque are lifelong friends, the kind of friends you have where you're like, "How did I even live my life without knowing you?" And when I say it's constant I mean it. For instance, I'm polyamorous. I have four partners, and one of my partners is actually a business partner too. So there's, like, no line dividing when we're discussing our personal stuff and when we're discussing burlesque stuff. The business part of it just weaves in and out. It's a really interesting life to live.

Pre-COVID, I was traveling across the country, performing in burlesque festivals or doing featured shows in other places. Last January, for instance, I went down to San Diego and was a featured performer for a burlesque troupe down there. It was really fun and really exciting. Afterward the organizers were saying to me, "Okay, in 2020 we're gonna have you back!" And I was like, "Oh, yeah! I'm here for it." Obviously, that didn't happen . . . Looking at my calendar and seeing all the stuff I had lined up for 2020 before COVID—that was really hard. But it happened.

COVID happened, so we had to pivot. It really did change the landscape of my work, especially my sex work. I'm a pro-domme sex worker and I work predominantly with queer femmes who want to do BDSM, want to do kink, but they don't trust their partners to do it; or they might have some hang-ups with BDSM and kink, so they come to me to help them through that. It's like equal parts happy fun time and equal parts therapy, you know? It's a very safe space to practice in and I get to decide who my clients are. I get to decide who I want to see and how that looks, how that works. It's a very niche market, but it's really therapeutic and healing for folks, and I like being able to provide that. But, of course, once COVID happened that made things very difficult, because you're in the business of touching people and now you can't touch people that way—it's not safe. Especially in those early days when we didn't know shit about shit . . . "How is this thing spreading? Is it jumping through masks?" We didn't know if it could even be done safely, and I couldn't take the risk. I got a kid at home.

Max: Let's talk about that a bit more. Could you put yourself back in that headspace and talk about what it was like for you as the reality of COVID-19 started to set in?

Mx. Pucks: Honestly, it's not even that hard to put myself back in that headspace, because Facebook has those "Memories" that pop up on your timeline . . .

Max: That's right! Those things always throw me for a loop, to be honest, because my sense of linear time is all fucked up now.

Mx. Pucks: Yeah, it's like I almost depend on Facebook Memories right now to help piece certain things together. Otherwise I'm just like, "What? What happened? Where are we?" This time last year, in February, we had a big show about to come up—I co-produced a show called "It's All for You: A Janet Jackson Review." All the acts were using Janet Jackson music and it was an all-people-of-color show. We had booked the show at this relatively large venue, so it was going to be a big leveling-up moment for the production company. At that point we had heard the whispers of COVID, but it hadn't really started to sink in yet, because we weren't really getting that much information, and we had no idea what was on the horizon . . . But yeah, February of 2020, there were a lot of things I was looking forward to. I had gotten accepted into the Utah Burlesque Festival, for instance. They were doing their very first burlesque festival and we were super excited about that. That was gonna be in March. Then, in May, I was supposed to be going to Panama for the Panama Burlesque Festival. Also, I was co-producing a festival that we were bringing to Seattle called "Fierce!" which is an all-queer burlesque festival—that was gonna happen in May too. That would have been the seventh year of the "Fierce!" festival. Every year they travel across the country and put this festival on in a different location, and I had actually petitioned to have the city of Seattle be the place where the 2020 festival would happen. I also had all these really cool side gigs coming up that I was really looking forward to. I was supposed to be doing a handfasting ceremony[10] last fall with one of my partners, who was turning into kind of a big deal, and that was really neat. So I was in a really interesting place in February of last year—looking forward, it just felt like 2020 was gonna be this weird year that would propel me forward as a burlesque performer and as a producer. And also, I was starting to find this nice little groove with my pro-domme stuff. It was a really cool place to be—you could kind of feel this vibration in the air, like something neat was gonna happen.

Then March happened . . . It was early March, I think. There was all these whispers about venues possibly having to close down and people were a little on edge. And my schedule for the first two weeks of March was really, really booked. I had so many gigs, like back-to-back-to-back gigs. The second-to-last gig I did before the shutdown was for a show here in Seattle called the "Sunday Night Shuga Shaq." It is produced by Ms. Briq House and Sin de la Rosa, who are just these two fantastic BIPOC burlesque babes, and it's an all-people-of-color burlesque show. That show's usually sold out—it's wild. It's not at all what you would think a burlesque show should be, but everything you kind of secretly hoped it would be. That night, when we were all getting ready, there was just this feeling in

10 Handfasting is a symbolic marriage ritual that has its origins in ancient Celtic culture. During the handfasting ceremony, the hands of the people getting married are carefully bound at the wrists with rope or cloth to symbolize the binding of their lives.

the air that, like, this could be it . . . at least for a while. And so, we all went out there and we just gave that audience everything we had. I performed a newer act that night—it's like a super classic burlesque act, which I don't typically do—and I got a standing ovation. I'd never, ever received a standing ovation before that. It was kind of a weird, magical night. Then, on March 10 . . . that was my last in-person gig. That was down in this town called Olympia, Washington. I remember talking to one of the producers of that show as we were getting ready and she said, "If you get any information about whether or not we can keep doing shows will you let me know?" And I was like, "Absolutely. Guess we'll have to see what the governor of Washington says . . ." I've gone down there and performed in Olympia several times, specifically with this group of producers, and their shows are always really wild—there's always a lot of people. But that night, for that show, the audience was about a third of the normal size. And I just knew that was the last time I was going to be on stage for a minute.

This is the real kicker . . . It was right around March 12–14 that shit really kicked off, right? That's when the world went to hell in a handbasket. New York was just like, "It's time to shut down." Then everyone started shutting down. Well, there was a burlesque festival happening in New York that weekend . . .

Max: Oh, Jesus . . .

Mx. Pucks: All these people had traveled from all over the country to be there. There was also a burlesque festival happening in Alaska. I just immediately went into panic mode thinking about all these people I love traveling all over the country as they're locking stuff down . . . "What's gonna happen?" And then this tragic thing starts happening: show after show after festival after festival starts canceling. You watch as people try to hold out like, "Maybe it could still happen. We could wait and see . . ." But, just like dominoes, one after another after another, everything got cancelled. After a while you didn't even want to be on Facebook anymore because there was gonna be news of another big cancellation.

I was supposed to produce this birthday show for Miss Indigo Blue, who is a burlesque legend in the making—she runs the Academy of Burlesque here in Seattle. And it was gonna be a *big* birthday show for her fiftieth birthday. So, obviously I wanted to do it because I really care about this person. And there was also that part of me that knew, like, "If I produce this show for her and I produce it well, everyone will know that I did that. And that's another step on this journey that I'm on to be, you know, an elite producer." But we had to cancel that show. We canceled all these things. That's when it really started to set in that . . . a lot of folks who heavily depend on their burlesque income are losing it. And then the anxiety sets in. Speaking of which, I remember that first full weekend after they started doing the lockdown stuff, because my partner was like, "We should do mushrooms! It'll be great." And I was like, "Sure." Bad idea. I cried every single tear I think I've ever had in my body that night—just broke down sobbing. All I could think was, "Burlesque as we know it is for-ever changed. There's no way around it, and I don't know what to do about it." And I'm not a person who likes feeling powerless at all. I don't like it. So then everyone was trying to figure out what to do, and some folks were like, "We should move to doing burlesque virtually." But I was like, "Ew, gross. I don't want to do that," mostly because all of the copyright laws are really wackadoo when stuff is online—they're not really straightforward about what you can and can't do. And when you try to get direct answers from these companies about how you can use this or that music, where you can use it, etc., it's a lot of running around. For instance, some of the earlier burlesque and drag shows were on Instagram Live and Facebook Live and those shows were getting booted, or they would just mute the music. On top of that, there didn't really seem to be a way to monetize that, which is why I was like, "So, y'all are just out here doing all that for free? Oh, no. No, thank you." I really was not trying to hear that noise at all. Then I got a message from a really good friend who used to live out here in Seattle. She's based in Florida now, and she was like, "Hey, let's do a digital burlesque show," and I said no. But then she said, "I got a live band now," and I was like, "Okay, I'm listening . . ." And so, in April, I helped put together this show that had a live band playing their own music. All of the burlesque acts were based off this band's music—they own their music, they gave us permission to use the music, so we did a virtual show through Zoom that way. And that's what I've been doing ever since: virtual shows through Zoom or another really cool platform called Crowdcast. It's kept me busy—I mean really busy. I created an online class for other producers to watch to assess whether or not they have what it takes to produce a virtual show. Basically, the class is meant to convince you not to do it [laughs]. That is how I wrote it. I'm just like, "You can jump off this train at any time. If you make it to the end, great." But yeah, I really pivoted very hard. Once I felt like I understood how the copyright stuff works and all of that I kind of pushed full steam into it. Now I probably produce a virtual show every other month. It's got its pluses and minuses. I mean, it's really cool to be able to produce a show in your pajamas . . .

Max: I mean, let's be honest: Being able to do any kind of work in your pajamas fucking rocks. [Laughs.]

Mx. Pucks: Right? I get to be business up top and below I'm wearing unicorn slippers and yoga pants, and that's really neat. You just kind of roll out of bed and there you are—you're in the space. Pivoting to virtual productions also means I've had to learn all kinds of cool stuff. I had to learn how to do video editing. I had no clue how to do that before the pandemic. I've been learning how to do lighting, etc. Now I'm like deeply, emotionally invested in backdrops [laughs]. I'm just like, "Ooh, that's a cool backdrop!" then I'll go buy tons of fucking fabric to make curtains and shit. And that's not . . . I wouldn't have ever expected that out of myself. When you're doing these kinds of productions you become your own set designer, your own director, etc. Basically, right now, people who are making and recording burlesque stuff—they're making, like, music videos, and it's really neat. It's a really cool thing that's happening. But not everyone has it in them. That's been a really painful thing to watch. A lot of really amazing burlesque performers are struggling with their sense of identity, because virtual performing is not at all a replacement for performing in front of a live audience. You don't have that energy, that power exchange that happens when you're giving them all of you on stage and they're giving you their attention, they're giving you their applause. It's very much a voyeur-and-exhibitionist type situation, and for a lot of burlesque folks that is why they're in it. Doing these virtual shows and pre-recorded acts doesn't give them the same high at all. It's actually more stress. And that lost sense of identity, that lost sense of self, goes even deeper. It really is kind of a fucked-up deal because, you know, you have a burlesque persona, everyone has a burlesque persona. For some people, their burlesque persona is a completely fabricated character, and that's really neat. For other folks, their burlesque persona is basically who they are in real life but turned up to eleven. And so, this identity crisis starts to emerge. It's like, "If I'm not this, what do I have? What am I?" I will say that Mx. Pucks A'Plenty is not a complete fabrication at all. Mx. Pucks A'Plenty is me. I already live life at about an eight or nine. Mx. Pucks A'Plenty just wears *a lot* more makeup and wears more rhinestones—that's about it. It's gotten to the point that when I hear my real name I am confused and flustered by it. When my legal name is used I'm just like, "Where's my mother? Where is she?" Cuz she is really the only person who calls me that . . . well, my mom and like one of my ex-husbands. And I don't want to deal with him, and I don't want to deal with her. So who is using my real name? Everyone calls me "Pucks," and I just have such an attachment to it. I'm Pucks and Pucks is me—it is what it is. I think that's why I haven't really suffered as much with this identity crisis, because Mx. Pucks was always me.

The cool thing about me is that I'm gonna complain the whole fucking time when something isn't going right, or isn't going the way I want it to, but as I'm complaining I'm also MacGyvering the fuck out of shit around me, you know? That's why I have a hard time with people who complain and don't do anything to fix their situation. Like, if you're gonna complain pick up these fucking sticks, because we're about to build some shit—let's do this. That's me. I'm gonna whine and complain and whine and complain, and then, when I'm done, I'll be like, "Alright, I fucking built a house, now get in it. Let's go." I had a really interesting conversation about resilience with a good friend of mine. The thing is, I would prefer not to have to be resilient. I would prefer not to need to have this strength. I would prefer to just be very vulnerable and have people do everything for me—that would be really fucking delightful. But that's not the reality, right? Not at all. I *have* to show up, because if I don't show up it's not gonna get done. And by "it" I mean life. My life won't get done if I don't show up for it. I can't ask someone else to show up for my life for me. And COVID has definitely put a really big spotlight on that. If I don't make it happen, I don't eat, my kid doesn't eat.

A lot of theater folks and performing arts folks got really shafted on a lot of the aid that the government initially put out when they realized,

"Oh, fuck, this COVID stuff is getting really out of control." We talked a lot about "essential workers," but we didn't really think about what it would look like for all the other folks out there who were no longer able to go into work. For instance, I didn't qualify for a lot of the grants and stuff like that. I didn't even qualify for unemployment . . .

Max: Ugh, what the hell?

Mx. Pucks: Right? It was just like, "Oh, cool. So what am I supposed to do now?" And all I had was virtual burlesque, so I had to make it work. But then I realized my production company qualifies for grants, so I applied for every grant that I possibly could—because, again, we're fiscally sponsored, so we're technically a 501(c)(3). It was because of those grants that I was able to redistribute some money to people who really needed it. By doing these shows I was able to pay burlesque performers, the most marginalized folks. I was able to put money in their pockets. It was like, "Look, I can't just write you a blank check, because I don't have that kind of money. But if you come do this show I can get you paid, and I can get you paid well." That was the most heartbreaking part. I knew I'd figure out my situation somehow, but it was really hard watching my other artist friends not being able to make ends meet, worrying about money, worrying about this or that, because you want to help them and you're like, "Oh, my God. What are we going to do?" This was one way I could go to people and say, "I know it's a tall order to ask you to put together a burlesque act, but if you *can* I can get you money. I can put money in your pocket." And I got a lot of shit for it in the beginning. Folks were just like, "We don't know why you're doing this. We don't understand." If you can't understand that this is the only way I can give people money, then it's not worth having the conversation . . . It's thankless sometimes.

You know, there are people in the burlesque community who are not fans of mine, who do not like me at all, because I'm very vocal. When I see stuff that isn't right, when I see stuff that lacks integrity, I call it out very quickly. For me, it's best to just rip the Band-Aid off and do it. I'm always pushing for honest and frank conversations within the burlesque community. Stop saying that "burlesque is for everybody," for instance, when you're only casting skinny people on your show, or you're only casting

White or White-passing burlesque performers. If you're going to say that burlesque is for everybody, then you should show that in what you're producing and what you're putting out there.

Max: Just from talking to friends and other folks I'm connected to, I know how big of a problem the unemployment system has been for so many people like yourself. My parents had a hell of a time getting on unemployment. Practically everyone I know told me horror stories about being on the phone for hours and waiting to get through to somebody, if they got through to anybody. But, like you said, it's been even worse for sex workers and artists and a lot of people who just didn't qualify because of their job or immigration status or whatever, and where were they supposed to turn? It was just like, "Well, sorry, you're on your own." And so, because of that, you started seeing more people turning to making money online, like y'all did with the virtual burlesque shows. And you had a lot of folks who rushed to sites like OnlyFans to do online sex work, because they could make money there when they couldn't get aid from the government, right? It sounds like a lot of artists in the burlesque industry were doing that as well?

Mx. Pucks: Absolutely. It was probably around April-ish that, all of a sudden, a bunch of folks were talking about starting OnlyFans accounts, and I remember being very cranky about it, because a lot of those folks are the same ones who were saying, "I'm not a stripper," or just generally trying to distance themselves from sex workers. And I was just like, "What do you think OnlyFans is? That's a form of sex work. What are you even talking about?" The hypocrisy of it was very difficult for me. Again, integrity is something that really matters to me, so it really pissed me off. Also, the part of it that *really* pissed me off was that I knew all of these folks who had OnlyFans before all this stuff began, who worked really fucking hard to build up their clientele to the point that they could use OnlyFans as their main money-making venture. For a lot of people OnlyFans is their livelihood. Now that market's fucking flooded. There was only so much money to go around in the first place, but now there are way more mouths to feed. So, it's like we're robbing from each other. Sure, this person who didn't have an OnlyFans before is now making X amount of money, but the person who was making their money on OnlyFans before that saw a cut of like 25 to 50 percent of their income? It's very . . . it's really weird.

I don't fault anyone for having an OnlyFans. I think it's great. I've seen some really dope OnlyFans—and, as a person who just loves porn in general, I think OnlyFans is a fairly ethical way to consume porn. I'm all about the ethical consumption of porn. I want to make sure that the performers in porn get paid, and I want them to get paid well. If I know that the way I'm sourcing this porn is ethical and that the person on film is getting the majority of that money, then . . . I don't know, it's like when I come I feel like I'm an angel who got my wings. I did my part [laughs]. It's just like, "Man, that was an ethical orgasm . . ." [Laughs.]

Max: [Laughs.] "I've done my good deed for the day . . ."

Mx. Pucks: Right? And that feels good! Nobody wants to have a guilty orgasm. So, that's a very interesting part of the OnlyFans conundrum for me. But, again, the main thing I couldn't stomach was all the folks who were very anti-sex-worker or very anti-stripper—"I'm not a stripper, blah, blah"—and who now have OnlyFans. I'm just sitting here like, "There's not enough weed in the world for me to process the hypocrisy of that . . . like, at all."

Max: [Laughs.]

Mx. Pucks: I'm not on OnlyFans—that's not where I need to be. And that's not me saying, "Oh, I'm too good for OnlyFans." No, that market is saturated. I don't need to be there taking money away from other people. For me the question was, "What am I gonna do with all this sex knowledge that I have? Where's all that gonna go?" So I started a podcast with a good friend of mine who is a sex therapist and sex educator. It's called *SexualiTea SEA*, and I'm really proud of it. It's really good. That is where all of that sexy sauciness went—it went into building this podcast. We have a Patreon set up for it and everything. So that's the route I ended up taking. It was just like, "I'ma keep my ass off OnlyFans so that the folks there can make their money. That's where they need to be, and this is where I'm going to be." It's just a different journey.

So, yeah, I've been doing the virtual burlesque shows, then I've been doing the podcast, and the podcast is going really well. It's really cute and funny and it's really educational, really insightful, and very candid . . . that's just the kind of person that I am. My co-host—they're more of a Type-A personality. I am definitely not an A-type personality [laughs], so we're really good foils for each other on the podcast. And we've been interviewing a lot of burlesque people on the podcast too. It seems like every burlesque person I know, they got another hook, they got another hustle, they got another thing going on, and a lot of burlesque people are also sex and sexuality educators. It's been really fascinating to talk to folks I know from burlesque on the podcast and explore this other part of their world. It doesn't make a whole lot of money, but it makes enough to pay for itself. At the end of the day, that's pretty great.

Max: Even just deciding to start a podcast, though . . . that kind of goes back to what we were talking about before, right? In so many ways COVID-19 kind of forced us all into different stages of evolution. It forced us to find our creative outlets, to find ways to stay connected with each other, because we *need* that connection. If we have to socially distance we still have to find creative ways to maintain our sense of community and togetherness. And, of course, COVID forced many of us to locate or create new ways of getting income. I guess all of that has just got me thinking about where things are gonna be if and when we ever get this "return to normalcy," you know? In that vein, I wanted to round things out by asking what you think the future is for burlesque and for burlesque workers like yourself after COVID?

Mx. Pucks: I would say that my life pre-COVID was not one that I'd like to return to. Yeah, I had a lot of things lined up for 2020 and it was gonna be great, but my living situation wasn't ideal. I was making some income doing burlesque and doing production stuff, but I was really overwhelmed and always felt like I was working hard but not really getting a chance to play hard. And of course I was still fighting with other producers in the industry about, like, their shows not being diverse enough. I have no desire for things to go back to how they were pre-COVID—it wasn't a great place to be.

When we got into that May time frame . . . that's when you could feel something changing. That's when the video that really woke a lot of people up started going around. That video of George Floyd with a cop's knee in the back of his neck . . . If it wasn't for COVID that wouldn't have even been a blip on the screen. The murder of George Floyd would have just been some story that got buried on people's newsfeeds. I think . . . COVID made people aware. COVID made people wake up. It pulled you out of that day-to-day grind. We were all cogs in the capitalist machine before, but COVID sort of stopped that machine for a lot of us, at least long enough for the fog to start lifting. And after the initial novelty of quarantine wore off, after you played all the online games you could find, folks started having these moments like, "Well, I guess I should do some self-reflection or something." And seeing this man die on camera with a knee on the back of his neck—I think that sparked a lot of self-reflection. We saw our nation just rise up and say, "No, we don't want this. Black lives actually *do* matter." And people were so hyper-focused on the issue because a lot of folks didn't have work, right? We were dredged in existential dread about what we were gonna do for money and how we were gonna get by, but we saw how many others were in the same boat. This was a moment for folks to take a break from thinking about themselves and start thinking about others—to see ourselves as more of a collective and take care of each other, which is really beautiful. And that's why I think you see a lot of mutual aid efforts popping up everywhere, which is amazing. Speaking of mutual aid, I was at the protests that became the Capitol Hill Occupied Protest. I used what little I had as a burlesque producer and performer in the Seattle area to start fundraisers and raise money to bring supplies up to the medics who were up on the hill for the protests, to make sure they had water, masks, hand sanitizer, umbrellas, cots—all kinds of things. I think I ended up raising somewhere around $2,000 or $3,000 to make sure there were supplies up there. There was a small contingent of Seattle-based burlesquers who were out there on the front line during the protests. There were other burlesque babes who became trained street medics so they could help rinse people's eyes out when they got tear-gassed. I was there the night the Seattle police abandoned the East Precinct. I made a guy wrestle a microphone away from these two guys who were arguing onstage, and I went up there and spoke to around one-thousand people who were there that night . . . Burlesque is political. It always has been. And I feel like I'd be doing a huge disservice if I didn't use my voice to fire other people up and to get people to stand up for what they believe in.

When I look at the future of burlesque . . . I am excited for all the things that I'm working on and for all these amazing people I get to work with. I'm also a little depressed because there are folks out there who didn't learn shit during this whole fucking time. And I'm just like, "You have to actively choose to be ignorant if you're not taking any lessons from this pandemic. You must be allergic to learning." And so . . . I know there's going to be some business-as-usual bullshit when the world opens back up. But I've been sitting here, doing my thing, working with people, talking to people, raising money, doing this, doing that—I've been very quiet about some things, but I've been pretty loud about others. I am hoping that the folks I see who move in this industry with integrity . . . I'm hoping that our voices will be much louder than the voices of these ignorant folks who still want to debate things like whether or not cultural appropriation is a thing. I am past the point of debating and arguing with folks about things like privilege, racial discrimination, police brutality, institutional oppression—all of that. There's no debate: it's fact. When people are choosing to be ignorant about facts, when you get into this "alternative facts" situation, it's just like . . . I feel like arguing with folks about this kind of thing is pointless. I also feel like I'm fighting below my weight class, you know? It's almost like pushing a kid down as an adult—that's how I look at it. Trying to fight with someone who is outclassed for this conversation is actually cruel of me. They got to learn that shit on their own—I'm not here to pass out free education. I feel that way when folks don't quite understand burlesque, too. I don't give out free education. And I don't give out free education about sex work or anything like that. Pay me for my time and pay me what I'm worth.

I'm definitely looking forward to what is on the other side of a post-COVID life. Part of that, though, also involves recognizing that this whole thing was so fundamentally fucked up. Like, everything the United States did or didn't do to handle COVID was just a debacle from the word "Go." Unfortunately, it sounds like COVID is probably here to stay. Like the flu, it'll be here . . . it's just part of our reality now, and that's the most horrifying part. When the world does open back up all these other countries that did all the things they could do to protect themselves will still be dealing with COVID, because countries like ours had the opportunity to tackle this thing globally, to eradicate it—we had the opportunity to make the buck stop here, but mediocrity won. And it wasn't just all Trump. I didn't want to talk about Trump, but I guess I will really quick. It's just like how folks want to say that Trump is responsible for all the racism we see in this country. No, no, no, it was already there. He just fanned the flames. I don't think he's actually a very intelligent human being at all, but he's a charismatic human being. He is the poster child of mediocrity and failing upwards, right? There are so many cishet White men for whom Trump is a symbol of failing and still getting ahead without any repercussion for those failures and what they leave in their wake. If that's not an apt metaphor for the crumbling of our society I don't know what is.

But I still have hope. I hope that the other side of COVID involves us really doing the work to end some of this institutional racism and all the other things that are actually holding *all* of us back. I tell folks all the time, "White supremacy hurts everybody, even White people." It's a very cruel device that is used to keep all of us separated from each other—and that's the goal. That's always been the goal. If you keep all these people fighting over one fucking cookie while you got the eleven other cookies from the dozen, you win. You don't want all those people fighting over that one cookie to be like, "Wait a minute . . . all the cookies are over *there*. We should all team up and get the cookies." I think, once we can work through this bullshit and figure that out, our country's gonna be in a lot better place.

About the Author

Maximillian Alvarez is a writer and editor based in Baltimore. His work has been featured in outlets including *The Nation, In These Times, Boston Review, The Baffler, The New Republic, Protean* magazine, and the *Chronicle of Higher Education*. He is currently the editor in chief of The Real News Network and the host of *Working People*, a podcast about the lives, jobs, dreams, and struggles of the working class today.